30 Things Future Dads Should Know About Pregnancy

To the at-home dads who prove every day that the true measure of a dad is in the size of his heart. (Daddyshome, www.daddyshome.org)

30 Things Future Dads Should Know About Pregnancy

Hogan Hilling

TRADE PAPER PRESS

Turner Publishing Company
200 4th Avenue North • Suite 950
Nashville, Tennessee 37219
(615) 255-2665

www.turnerpublishing.com

30 Things Future Dads Should Know About Pregnancy

Library of Congress Cataloging-in-Publication Data
Hilling, Hogan.
 30 things future dads should know about pregnancy / Hogan Hilling.
     p. cm.
 ISBN 978-1-59652-592-4
1. Fatherhood. 2. Motherhood. 3. Pregnancy. 4. Wives--Psychology. I. Title. II. Title: Thirty things
future dads should know about pregnancy.
 HQ756.H554 2010
 306.874'2--dc22
                                    2010025775

Printed in China

10 11 12 13 14 15 16 17—0 9 8 7 6 5 4 3 2 1

"There is a choice you have to make in everything you do. And you must always keep in mind the choice you make, makes you."

–Anonymous

Contents

Introduction

Introduction

When a wife asks her husband to conceive a baby, almost every husband is willing to become a dad and help his wife fulfill her lifelong dream: to be a mom. Once a wife announces her pregnancy, it is a very joyous occasion. However, with the blissful confirmation of the unborn baby, a husband also inherits a list of challenging issues with his future role as a dad that he may be unaware of or afraid to address. I wrote this book to explore many of these common issues a future dad will need to tackle and resolve during his wife's pregnancy.

The information in this book is based on my personal experiences as a dad of three pregnancies and interaction with a melting pot of dads I've had the pleasure of meeting and networking with since 1992.

My debut as a dad began in 1987 after my wife, Tina, announced her pregnancy. In 1992 I cofounded the Fathers Network of Orange County, a support group for fathers of children with special needs. Two years later, I was hired as a consultant and instructor for Boot Camp for New Dads (BCND) in Irvine, California. Today, BCND is a nationally recognized program that provides classes for expectant dads in hospitals across the U.S. In 2002, I founded Proud Dads, Inc., a consulting firm to improve support services for dads.

What I have learned through my experience is that dads want to do their part to be involved in every aspect of the pregnancy. But they feel just as unprepared, confused, detached from the unborn baby, and frustrated as I did during all three of my wife's pregnancies.

And just like me, their disappointments stemmed from the lack of attention in addressing an expectant dad's concerns and the lack of resources and support services for expectant dads.

Unfortunately, very little progress has been made in the last twenty years to accommodate, service, and engage dads during the pregnancy. Nevertheless, don't let that discourage your efforts and desire to be a great dad. It didn't dampen my spirit—it motivated me to write this book. Furthermore, the issues remain the same. Here are some of the issues and anxieties dads have shared with me.

"I'd like to do my part to be an involved dad during the pregnancy, but how can I if access to resources and support services for new dads is limited and not readily accessible in the same way it is for new moms?"

"I'd like to be valued as an equal partner. But that's not possible when most of the attention is focused on servicing my wife's concerns and needs."

"Okay, so my wife is the one who is pregnant. But that shouldn't devalue my role as a new dad.

One minute I'm a new dad. Next thing I know I've been demoted by the childbirth instructor to coach, partner, helper, or significant other. I thought I was the dad?"

"Every time my wife has a concern and needs support or information about her pregnancy, it's only a phone call or stone's throw away from her. But when I need help or support, it's like looking for a needle in a haystack."

"Why is most of the information about pregnancy written for Venusians in their native language? Any of these childbirth instructors know how to speak Martian?"

If you can relate to any of these dads, then this book is for you. If you want to learn how to be the best dad you can be during your wife's pregnancy, then you will appreciate what this book has to offer. Here is how *30 Things* can help.

A man is at a huge disadvantage when he enters the world of pregnancy in the same way a woman was when she decided to enter the world of corporate America's good ole boy's club in the 1970s. Plenty of evidence proves that today's world of pregnancy is heavily biased toward moms. The bias exists in our culture due to the misconceptions about men as inept caregivers, and the lack of effort and funding by the medical health industry, government agencies, and corporate America to provide identifiable resource and support services for dads comparable to those for moms. A trip to the local bookstore will also confirm that books to help prepare women for motherhood dominate the pregnancy shelves. The odds that the pregnancy world will level the playing field any time soon are slim because any change or adjustment in the current operating system might be viewed as detrimental to motherhood.

Despite this bias, this book will help you increase the chances for success in fulfilling your role as a new dad during the pregnancy. It will teach you how to comfort your pregnant wife and earn brownie points from her; boost your confidence in your quest to be a great dad; diplomatically navigate your way through a mother's turf and the medical staff; deal with your pregnant wife's mood swings; establish your value as a new dad; manage your new life as a family man; overcome the anxieties about being in the delivery room; tackle sensitive issues like sex, bonding with the unborn baby, and finances; and find viable resources and support services.

Becoming a new dad is a huge responsibility, and most men's greatest fear about fatherhood is that of the unknown. No man likes to go into unfamiliar territory unprepared. I hope the information in this book will help you become better equipped and educated than I and other dads were when we ventured into the world of fatherhood.

Good luck, and remember to enjoy the pregnancy journey!

The 30 Things

~ 1 ~

You're not having a baby,
you're having a
third person

─ 1 ─

You're not having a baby, you're having a third person

When a man decides to marry a woman, he is gaining a wife, but he is also bringing a second person into his life. Well, the same is true when a wife and husband decide to conceive a baby. As they get caught up in the romance of having a baby, oftentimes they don't realize that they are bringing a third person into their life.

While that sounds obvious, what I mean is that having a baby will affect your relationship with your wife much more than, say, getting a dog or cat. A baby is not a pet you acquire. A baby is a human being that grows into a child, a teenager, and then an adult.

Once a husband agrees to have a baby, as a new dad, he will have to make adjustments in his life and take on new responsibilities and adapt to new situations just as he did during his transition from singlehood to husbandhood. The baby will change the dynamics of a new dad's life just as his fiancé did when she became a wife. A new dad's relationship with his wife will also change because both will take on different, additional roles, a wife as a mom, and husband as a dad. But this change is actually a good thing, because there's more to life than self-indulgence. Once the pregnancy has been confirmed, mom and dad now collaborate to care for a third person—the baby.

The pregnancy will be a joyous time to celebrate and enjoy with family and friends. But the reality is that whatever life a new dad was accustomed to before the pregnancy will now change dramatically. How? The baby will affect how a new dad will communicate, make decisions, and interact with his wife. During the pregnancy, a new dad may not stay out late with friends, or sleep in until eleven in the morning cuddling with his wife and wondering what he'll do the rest of the day. There will be new concerns and lengthy discussion with your wife on topics such as which hospital to choose to deliver the baby, what type of childbirth classes to attend, which birth method to choose, how to address financial concerns, what books to read, what name for the baby you'll choose, and what your role in the delivery room will be. As you read through this book, I'll cover many more issues a new dad will have to address and discuss with his wife and mother-to-be.

Remember that adage "Two's company; three's a crowd"? Well, it is not necessarily true that a group of two people is more comfortable than a group of three, but a new dad may feel like it after the baby arrives. The difference is that the baby had received an invitation and will become a permanent member of a new family.

Three is good company for now. That is until a new dad decides to bring a fourth, fifth, or sixth person into his life. But for now I wish you the best of luck with the new baby—a.k.a. the third person.

— 2 —

She's the one who's pregnant

− 2 −
She's the one who's pregnant

As much as some people joke about it or want you to believe a dad becomes pregnant just by the very nature of a mom being pregnant, the truth is that a dad cannot be pregnant. It is physically and emotionally impossible. Pregnancy is a beautiful, amazing miracle to be cherished, so let's not taint it by acknowledging that dad is also pregnant. The art of being pregnant belongs to a mom; it's what makes her special. Her body was beautifully and specifically designed to grow and nurture a fetus into a baby and then deliver it. Although news of the pregnancy is an exciting moment for a new dad, the reality is that a new dad will never be able to have any real perspective of what it is like to be pregnant.

Except for some temporary bags under a new dad's eyes, he gets to look pretty much the same for nine months. Although Birthways, Inc. designed a weighted vest called the Empathy Belly that allows a new dad to experience pregnancy firsthand and gain a physical understanding of what it feels like to be pregnant, the $649 vest is disingenuous. No amount of money or device will ever help a man realize or experience the discomfort of being pregnant because any time he feels uncomfortable wearing it, he can take it off. An Empathy Belly also can't emulate the other physical changes to a woman's body, like swollen legs and feet, increase in breast size and weight, constipation, heartburn, leg cramps, and stretching of skin. Then, of course, there will be the expansion of the cervix to deal with during labor and delivery. The list goes on and on.

Even if a dad were to wear the vest for nine months, all it really does is help a man feel what it's like to be twenty-five to thirty-five pounds heavier.

Pregnancy is physically exhausting, but it's nothing like carrying thirty-five pounds of equipment during a military training exercise in the middle of the jungle or desert. Pregnancy is a nine-month, 24/7 gig with no rest for the wicked. An expectant mom does not sleep well, either, because her body is constantly working to nourish her and the baby. Not only is her body growing, but so is the baby's body. The pregnant mom's body needs to add plenty of fluids and tissue to keep the baby alive. A pregnant women needs to gain an additional four pounds of blood, to say nothing of other fluids, breast tissue, and of course, some stores of fat to produce milk. No matter how well an expectant mom exercises and eats, her body will change, and she will gain weight. Some women's bodies change drastically, others not so much. Some women accept and handle the weight gain with ease. If your wife does, consider yourself lucky, because few take the change lightly.

Pregnancy can also be emotionally exhausting and bring out the worrywart in a new mom. The overwhelming responsibility of carrying the baby can induce a great deal of anxiety to which a dad cannot relate. A new mom has the added pressure of worrying about the baby's health. She has to be conscious of her diet because anything she consumes can directly affect the baby's development. A new mom may also have a level of concern that a new dad may not have about a miscarriage or the child being born with a deformity or disability. Nevertheless, it is also not possible for a woman to empathize with the emotions a man experiences during pregnancy. (I think it is important and beneficial to share this perspective with your wife, and we'll cover that in Chapter 24.)

As a new dad in 1987, I knew Tina was the one who was pregnant, but I took her for granted. I naturally assumed that Tina was aware of the serious nature of the pregnancy and the overwhelming sense of duty she was about to undertake just because she was a woman. I thought Tina had the pregnancy under control. And she did everything to make it appear that way. I didn't consider that this was her first time and that she was just as new to being pregnant as I was to being a dad. I was ignorant to all the information about pregnancy that I have described in the previous paragraphs. To paraphrase Prissy in *Gone With the Wind,* I didn't know nothin' about being pregnant. To say I didn't fully appreciate Tina being pregnant is an understatement.

As you embark on your journey as a new dad, please don't take your wife for granted, and show her some respect by acknowledging that she is the one who is pregnant.

— 3 —

Pregnancies sometimes do not end with babies

− 3 −

Pregnancies sometimes do not end with babies

What I'm going to talk about next is not given much attention in the best-selling pregnancy books that a new dad or mom is probably reading. Many pregnant couples avoid discussing the issue because it is a frightening thought.

Nevertheless, a new dad needs to consider the likelihood of his wife's pregnancy terminating, or having to be terminated, for natural reasons. The statistics show that between ten and twenty-five percent of all clinically recognized pregnancies end in miscarriage (also known as "spontaneous abortion"). The odds increase as a woman ages.

"Clinically recognized" means a pregnancy has been confirmed by a doctor, so there may be more pregnancies lost by women who haven't yet had their first OB-GYN appointment. In fact, many women who have miscarriages experience what's called a "chemical pregnancy": a pregnancy that is lost so quickly after the implantation that the woman may not even know she's pregnant, and may not notice much difference in time or symptoms between the pregnancy loss and her normal period. Most miscarriages occur in the first trimester of pregnancy, and in hospital emergency rooms, women with first trimester bleeding from this are a common sight.

If a troubled pregnancy continues, though, a woman may not know anything is wrong until she gets to the doctor and an ultrasound is performed. During an ultrasound, the doctor will be able to tell if there is a heartbeat or not, or if the pregnancy has been implanted in the wrong place. Those symptoms will tell the doctor if one of the two most common reasons for pregnancy loss has occurred: blighted ovum, and ectopic pregnancy.

A blighted ovum occurs when fertilization of the egg results in growth of tissue, but a fetus does not develop. Many times, a doctor will suggest the woman have a "D & C" (dilation and curettage), which removes the placental tissue and other endometrial material, since waiting for the tissue to be expelled naturally may take a couple of weeks. (A similar but less common condition is a "molar" pregnancy, which results in abnormal tissue growth, and is the result of a genetic abnormality.)

With an ectopic pregnancy (also called a tubal pregnancy), fertilization occurs, but the egg implants itself in the wrong place, usually in the fallopian tube. Such a pregnancy must be medically terminated, usually by surgery, because neither the fetus nor the mother can survive if it continues. Ectopic pregnancies become extremely painful by the time the fetus has grown to the size of the fallopian tube— there will be no mistaking your wife's need for a trip to the doctor's office or emergency room once an ectopic pregnancy reaches this point.

Here's what a new dad can do with the unpleasant information about a miscarriage. First, recognize that it could happen. By outlining the statistics and the types of miscarriage, I'm trying to make it clear that, especially for a new dad and mom in their thirties, trying to conceive a baby may require a few tries, even if there aren't problems with fertility. It is in a new dad and mom's best interest to be aware of the high rates of miscarriage so they can be prepared to deal with the news of a miscarriage and the grieving period that will follow. Even if the pregnancy was unplanned, losing a baby is hard.

News of the miscarriage may be even harder if you opted not to tell anyone about the pregnancy for the first trimester. Grieving in private is very difficult—everyone needs support when faced with a tough loss. Nevertheless, a new dad and mom will need to be prepared to talk about their loss with trusted loved ones or a therapist. This is not an appropriate time for a new dad to stuff his emotions as it will lead to trouble down the road. Yes, a new mom needs to take care of her needs, especially if she is laid up after a surgical procedure, and if she looks to be suffering more than her husband, he needs to be there to support her. However, a new dad must make a space for his own grief and find someone he can trust to confide in. Being a dad will have its own challenges later down the road, and a new dad needs to take care of himself emotionally so he can be strong for those times.

Another helpful tip is to recognize that some people don't start grieving right away. If a new mom seems philosophical and strong at the time she finds out she's miscarrying, don't think, "Well! That's that, then." The subconscious usually does not react quickly, so if in a week or two, your wife falls apart for no apparent reason, keep in mind that she is probably grieving the lost pregnancy. A husband may even want to mark "check in on wife" on the calendar for two weeks after receiving the news.

Here are some do's and don'ts for talking to a new mom about pregnancy loss:

- *Don't* blame it on her. Pregnancies are lost all the time, and a new dad can't attribute it to his wife riding a bike, taking the wrong kind or not enough vitamins, traveling, et cetera. Leave diagnoses to the doctor.
- *Don't* take the blame. A new dad may experience feelings of letting his wife down or feeling responsible in some way. View this unfortunate situation as an act of nature and not something done to contribute to the miscarriage.
- *Don't* classify a D & C or surgery to remove an ectopic pregnancy as an elective abortion. Do allow a new mom and the doctor to decide whether a medical procedure can or should be performed to assist in pregnancy termination.
- *Do* accept that the feelings of loss and grief are normal.
- *Do* remind yourselves that now you know you can conceive.
- *Do* tell loved ones about the loss so they can support you.

- *Do* make time for your own grief.
- *Do* consider counseling.

Most pregnancies don't result in miscarriages. Nevertheless, it is important for a new dad to be prepared if it happens to his wife.

— 4 —

Make time to be involved with the pregnancy

– 4 –

Make time to be involved with the pregnancy

In Chapter 2, I noted that a new mom is the one who is pregnant, not the dad. Yes, a new dad should defer to the new mom regarding her body, her physical safety and comfort, and her feelings that may swing from joy to despair. That's one way to be involved: to be there for her, to support her in a hands-on way during the ups and the downs.

There's plenty a new dad can do, and should do. A new dad will be there during conception, so he should be there during every stage of the pregnancy. The mom is the lifeblood and incubator for the baby, so when a new dad takes care of the mom's needs, he is also taking care of the baby's needs. This will be a new dad's opportunity to show off and practice his nurturing skills on his wife and adjust to treating her as the mother of the baby. (As a new dad will see, the relationship he will have with the baby's mother will be different than the husband-wife relationship.) These skills a new dad demonstrates will also help his wife gain confidence in his ability to nurture and care for the baby after birth. Therefore, it is important to be an active husband and dad during the pregnancy.

So, for starters, the most important thing you can do is encourage your wife to call you at work anytime she feels the need to talk to you about her feelings. Now, I know what you're thinking. You don't want to be bothered at work. But take a moment to think how this kind gesture will benefit both of you. Your wife will love you for suggesting this because it will reassure her that you truly want to be involved in every aspect of the pregnancy. It will also assure her that she can count on you to be there for her whenever she needs you. This "knight-in-shining-armor" gesture will also strengthen your relationship with your wife and your bond with the new baby, and establish you, the dad (not her mom, sister, or other female friends) as the number one person to turn to for support. (You will see the significance of this in Chapter 14.) When she does talk to you on the phone, just listen and show some sympathy rather than give advice or try to solve her problems. For example, "Honey, I'm sorry you're having a rough day. I'll come home as soon as I can. I love you." That's all you have to say. On your way home, buy her some flowers to cheer her up.

The next thing you can do is show support for your wife by attending OB-GYN appointments. Although a doctor's appointment, in a new dad's eyes, may not seem or feel like an exciting event worth giving up time from work or fun with his friends, this will be the first true test of his commitment as an involved dad. If a new dad doesn't follow through now, he will have a more difficult time being there for mom and baby after the birth. A new dad should ask his wife to schedule the appointment during a time that is flexible with his work schedule.

For example, if the husband works an early shift, he can ask the wife to schedule the appointment later during the day, and vice versa if he works a late shift. A new dad can also take a two-hour lunch break and schedule an 11:00 A.M. or 1:00 P.M. appointment. This way he can still return to the office and continue with his work and fulfill his commitment to his employer.

An appointment with the doctor is a very exciting time for a mom, especially appointments with sonograms. Together a new dad and mom can get a view of the heartbeat and see a well-formed baby well enough to learn the baby's sex. When my sons were born, ultrasounds were amazing and novel. Today, they're standard—the novel technology is the 3-D ultrasound. Most dads I've spoken with noted that seeing the baby inspired them to want to do more for their wives. "I didn't realize how exciting a sonogram could be until I saw the baby. Seeing the baby made me feel more connected to it. It was one of those you-had-to-be-there moments. And I'm glad I was there!"

Next, consider participating in the purchase and setup of baby goods and furniture. I've told moms in my workshops that including dad with picking out a diaper bag and putting together baby furniture will make him more likely to invest time in becoming an involved dad. If a new dad has had a chance to become familiar with all of the baby paraphernalia, then it won't be foreign and baffling when he is faced with figuring it out after the baby is born. That way he can focus his time on fulfilling the baby's needs and enjoying the baby's company.

Another advantage of getting involved now is that a new dad will have some say in how things are established in his family. This can range from the trivial to the monumental. If a new dad helps pick out the diaper bag, he may not get stuck with the silky pink flowered one. Or a new dad can buy his and her diaper bags. In the doctor's office, a new dad's opinion can be beneficial in assessing any medical decisions. When purchasing furniture, a dad-to-be may be more aware of safety standards that a mom may overlook. And when it comes to finances, a dad can help a new mom keep her spending habits in check.

A new mom will also have less energy and limitations when it comes to cleaning the house. Dads shouldn't be shy about vacuuming and mopping floors, scrubbing the bathtub, dusting, or cooking a meal. It's also important for a new dad to get involved by practicing warming up bottles, buckling the car seat, shopping for diapers and baby food, and familiarizing himself with many of the other duties of caring for a baby. This way, after the baby's birth, mom and dad will work more efficiently as a team.

~ 5 ~

Bonding with an unborn baby can be difficult, and that's okay

─ 5 ─

Bonding with an unborn baby can be difficult, and that's okay

A dad can never match a mom's physical bond with an unborn baby for obvious biological reasons. While the physical connection mom has makes it easier for her to establish a relationship with an unborn baby, it doesn't mean a mom has an emotional advantage over a dad. The only real advantage a mom has is a head start. And there is plenty of time for a dad to make up that time.

There is an implied belief that bonding comes naturally for moms, but that is not true. It is not a given for them. Bonding is a process that takes time. It doesn't happen overnight and is not limited to happening within a certain time frame. That is because it involves relationship building between two persons, her and the unborn baby, the "third person" as noted in Chapter 1.

Bonding is also a work in progress. Just like a marriage, it takes work to overcome all the emotional issues that come with building an intimate relationship with another person.

When I first heard news that Tina was pregnant, I was happy, but I didn't feel an immediate connection to our unborn baby. Even though Tina and I planned the pregnancy, I had my doubts about being a dad. My heart really wasn't into being a dad, so bonding was difficult. I went along with the pregnancy just to please Tina. She wanted to be a mom so badly that I wanted it more for her than for me. Which raised the question, "How do I bond with an unborn baby I'm not one hundred percent sure I want to have in my life?" It's a tough question to answer, not only for a dad, but also for a mom. And this is especially true with an unplanned pregnancy.

Some new moms, even with a planned pregnancy, don't always feel immediate joy. Like new fathers, they are also overwhelmed with some level of fear, resentment, or regret. Sadly, these moms are also forced to mask the feelings and concerns they have about their struggle to bond with the unborn baby.

Some moms resent the unborn baby for what he or she has done to her body: "Our unborn baby felt more like an invader of my body and added weight I didn't want to carry around anymore." "With the morning sickness, growing pains, backache, and weight gain, the unborn baby felt more like a curse than a blessing."

Some moms feel forced into pregnancy: "I felt pressured to have a baby, mostly by my mom. During the pregnancy I felt as though my body had been hijacked at gunpoint. For a short time, I had reservations about having the baby but I didn't tell my husband."

Unfortunately for some moms, there is no mutual affection, and the pregnancy is just about survival. For these women, adoption or abortion is often the end result.

The baby's sex can also have an affect on the bonding process. If you wanted a boy and got a girl, or vice versa, you may not feel very excited, which is a common reaction from both parents. Therefore, you may experience a delayed reaction of jubilation. These are normal issues and concerns that new dads and moms have about bonding.

So how do you actually bond with your unborn baby once you have understood the importance of doing so and know you'll be bonding even if your child is thankless at first? I can sum it up in one word: contact. And I mean that it in the spiritual sense. Albeit indirect contact involves only two of the five senses—touch and sound—a dad can still bond with an unborn baby despite not being able to see it, smell it, or receive feedback. As I noted on ABC's *The Story of Fathers and Sons* documentary, "The father and child relationship is about the soul."

Touch involves the physical contact with your wife's tummy and the work and time you put into nurturing and caring for her, attending her doctor's appointments, completing household chores, and doing other pregnancy-related activities listed in Chapter 4. Every physical task a dad completes connects him closer to the unborn baby.

Sound involves vocal interaction like greeting the unborn baby (by name if you have one) when you come home from work, and having a conversation that can include speaking and answering for the baby, or singing to him. Discussing fatherhood issues with relatives, friends, neighbors, and other dads is also part of the bonding process.

Bonding with an unborn baby is also different than with human beings like your wife or friend: with them, there is tangible interaction and gratifying responses you can measure that come in the form of a kiss, handshake, smile, hug, or compliment. Not so with an unborn baby. However, as you will see after the birth, the bonding process doesn't stop, and you will continue to nourish the daddy bond with each day the baby grows. And in return, the two of you will build a long-lasting father and child relationship.

Now, I know what you're probably thinking: *I'm not comfortable with this mushy, touchy-feely stuff—it's unmanly.* No, it's not!

The most courageous and macho thing a man can do is to become an involved dad by bonding with his unborn baby (and wife), even if it means having to step out of his comfort zone. It's the only way to explore and reap the benefits of fatherhood—and the sooner, the better.

The last and most important piece of advice I would like to offer is to not compete with your wife's bonding. A mom's bond with a baby will be different than a dad's. Competing with mom will only create conflict and jealousy. Focus on what you can do as a dad to strengthen your bond with the unborn baby. The unborn baby will not appreciate it right away but will in the years to come. And as your bond with the baby strengthens, so, too, will your relationship with your wife.

~ 6 ~

Discover your greatest obstacle

- 6 -

Discover your greatest obstacle

After I wrote my first book, an interviewer asked, "What is the biggest challenge a man faces as a dad?" My answer? "His EGO," or Everyone's Greatest Obstacle.

Becoming a new dad is one of the proudest moments in a man's life. A new dad should feel and act proud. And it is important to establish a sense of self-confidence and absolute belief in your ability. However, there is a difference between pride and ego. Pride is a desire to be the best. Ego is thinking you are the expert and therefore above other people.

Fatherhood, like any profession, is a learning process: the more you learn, the more knowledgeable you become. When a dad feels he has learned enough and become an expert, his chances of success decrease. No matter how much you think you know, there will always be room for improvement.

One of the most common mistakes I see a man make is not seeking and accepting information from other people. This has a lot to do with most men being unwilling to admit that they don't know everything. Get over it! Don't let your ego stop you from learning.

As a new dad, you will meet many people who have more knowledge than you in all aspects of parenting. These people include doctors, nurses, childbirth instructors, breast-feeding consultants, counselors, relatives, friends, strangers, other dads, and yes, your wife. As I noted in Chapter 4 about nurturing your wife during her pregnancy, it is also important to nurture relationships with all the people you meet on your journey into fatherhood. Be open-minded to receiving their input, even if you initially disagree with their opinion. They, especially other dads, will be your best resource.

Another great resource is books on pregnancy and fatherhood. Make the time to browse through a selection of books. Don't read every page—you may not have enough time. However, if you are an avid reader, feel free to take in as much information as you like.

As a new dad, you will also make mistakes because you won't have the benefit of experience. You will be introduced to knowledge you are unaware of and will experience a little humility, which is okay. A lot of the information and environment will be foreign to you. Instead of pretending to know what is going on, feel free to admit that you don't know but want to learn. And don't be afraid to ask questions or seek advice. If you are in a childbirth class or doctor's office and don't understand something, ask for clarification. There is no such thing as a stupid question regarding fatherhood.

Don't attempt to take on fatherhood by yourself. Nobody succeeds in life without help from other people. (I'll elaborate on this in Chapter 14, "Ask for help and build a support network for your family.")

As you continue to read this book, you will find examples of how to keep your ego from getting in the way of being a good, involved husband and dad.

Bringing a human being into this world is a humbling experience. Stay humble as you continue your path into fatherhood, and you will increase your chances of succeeding in your newfound career as a dad.

Leave your ego here before turning the page.

— 7 —

Establish credibility as a dad by deferring to experts

Establish credibility as a dad by deferring to experts

In the 1950s there was a popular television show called *Father Knows Best.* It was about a wise family man and his common-sense wife. Whenever the kids needed advice, they deferred to their father. In the real world of parenting, however, it doesn't play out this way, especially during pregnancy. Instead the theme is "Father Knows Very Little."

Because a mom's perspective and input are rarely questioned, she can be very hard on her husband, the new dad. In the mom's defense, she has been indoctrinated with the notion that a man is clueless and inept when it comes to pregnancy (and parenting). After all, what does a man know about being pregnant? There are also the hormonal mood swings that a mom can't control. Therefore, a pregnant mom is oftentimes not in the mood to accept an opinion, advice, or a suggestion from her husband—even if he observes that something isn't right or well.

As your wife is struggling through the pregnancy, you may notice some things that she is not doing or is not aware of. You may notice a change in her eating habits and weight, as well as abnormal behavior in the way she is handling the pregnancy. Do not offer your opinion or advice. Instead, use my third-party rule. Take notes and keep a record of what you notice with the date and time. Next, call the childbirth instructor or doctor to express your concerns and share the notes with him or her.

Then, invite your wife to visit the doctor or call the childbirth instructor, or schedule an appointment for her. You can also have the doctor's receptionist call your wife to talk her into scheduling an appointment, or you can ask the childbirth instructor to call her and ask how she is doing. During the conversation the childbirth instructor can delicately bring up some of the concerns you noted about your wife.

The childbirth instructor can then provide her with some suggestions on how to resolve whatever issue she is dealing with.

The reality is that if the same message comes from a doctor and childbirth instructor, it will have more credibility, and your wife will be more apt to listen and accept the advice. Establishing a relationship with the doctors and childbirth instructors is also a great way to demonstrate your involvement as a husband and father, a relationship that will prove even more valuable for you after the baby is born.

As noted in the previous chapter, another way to gain credibility with your wife is to browse through books on pregnancy. (You'll also be busy reading or browsing through books on fatherhood.) If your wife is reading or recommends a book on pregnancy, browse through it when you can. Then select and bookmark a few topics in the book with post-it notes and use that information as a conversation piece. The effort alone will impress your wife and score you some huge brownie points. As you will read in Chapter 24 ("Encourage your wife to accept a dad's perspective"), this exercise will be significant in helping your wife accept and understand a dad's perspective.

— 8 —

Adjust to your wife's mood swings

— 8 —
Adjust to your wife's mood swings

Every husband is a victim of his wife's mood swings brought on by PMS. There is no way to avoid it and no place to hide from the barrage of uncontrollable outbursts or emotions that accompany PMS. Now add pregnancy in the mix, and suddenly you're dealing with PMS on steroids and heightened mood swings.

As a young adult I had only heard about PMS. I must plead ignorance. I never attempted to learn about it until after my marriage. If I had, I could have made my life a lot easier. So before I delve into how to handle your wife's PMS, let me provide a brief overview of it because I know most new dads don't quite understand the science behind it.

Premenstrual syndrome refers to a wide range of physical or emotional symptoms that typically occur about five to eleven days before a woman starts her monthly menstrual cycle. PMS and pregnancy have a range of identical symptoms because both are triggered by similar changes in a woman's hormone levels. Common PMS symptoms include depression, irritability, crying, oversensitivity, and mood swings. The most common physical symptoms are pain, fatigue, bloating, weight gain, acne, and breast tenderness. Just reading about the symptoms is exhausting; I can't imagine what it's like experiencing them.

During PMS, a woman's estrogen hormones can increase brain activity and overstimulate her to the point that she experiences out-of-control outbursts. Although women suffer physically and emotionally from PMS, men also suffer emotionally and usually become the verbal punching bag. And more often than not, women deliver a sucker punch. Women also don't know when the PMS kicks in, so it's not like they're sucker punching men on purpose. And after they've yelled at their men, they feel guilty about it. It's a vicious cycle that can wear down even the toughest of men.

It would be nice to have some kind of warning signal so husbands know when to avoid their wives or prepare to deal with their symptoms. Maybe someone can invent a mood ring or device that gives men a PMS alert. The latter, however, may become as annoying as the PMS. But even when you know the punch is coming, there is no easy way to deal with it.

There is treatment available to relieve some symptoms of PMS, including exercise, diet, prescribed medication, and professional intervention. But there is no cure. Trust me, women (and men) wish there was.

Women, however, have no control of PMS just as men don't have full control of their penis's blood flow. And men can't relate to PMS just as women can't relate to MSB (see Chapter 12). Although there is nothing a husband can do about PMS, he can change the way he reacts to it.

The key is to focus not on the PMS but on the mood swings that follow. A woman's mood swings develop not just because of PMS and its symptoms but also from constant stress of life, the pregnancy, and wondering when the next set of PMS symptoms will take over her mind and body.

Here is my top ten list of suggestions to deal with your wife's PMS. How you implement these depends on your wife's personality and relationship you have with her. What will work with one of your wife's emotional tirades may not work with another one. So be prepared to make adjustments along the way.

1. Don't take what she says personally. You will need to quickly learn how to develop a thick skin.
2. Don't dismiss her actions or blame them on PMS. That may only make her more upset and add fuel to the fire.
3. Tell her you understand why she is upset and

ask what you can do for her. If she offers a suggestion or orders you to do something, even if you disagree and think she is being too critical, do it exactly the way she tells you.

4. Keep a cool head and bite your tongue. Sometimes it's best not to say anything or try to solve her problem.

5. Let her vent. Sometimes she'll just need to let off some steam.

6. Don't hold a grudge. Whatever she says to you take with a grain of salt. Sticks and stones will break your bones but her irrational tirades will never hurt you.

7. A simple hug or holding of her hand may suffice. However, if your wife is sensitive to touch, affection may not work.

8. Humor is another way to counteract your wife's verbal assault. If you can laugh it off, she may laugh it off with you. Here is my favorite PMS story a dad, Jeff, shared with me. At the time, Jeff had four daughters be-

tween the ages of twelve and eighteen. Jeff suggested to his wife, Connie, that he install five flagpole brackets in front of his house and select a colored flag to identify her and each of their daughters. Before he returned home from work, Connie was to place the colored flag or flags identifying whom Jeff should avoid or be aware of upon entering the house. If all five flags were out, he would keep on driving. Jeff and Connie never followed through with the idea. Nevertheless, this was Jeff's way of using humor to deal with a difficult situation.

9. Talking to other dads about your pregnant wife's PMS difficulties can help you feel like you're not the only one dealing with them. Sometimes you also need to vent and release your frustration about your wife's behavior.

10. If none of these suggestions work, you may need to seek professional help.

All of these point to you giving her the right-of-way with her feelings. She's the one who's pregnant. Let her feel any way she wants to about it, and let her change her mind about her feelings often. Be aware that she is not going to love or hate every minute of the pregnancy, and that her feelings of the pregnancy in retrospect may be very different than her current feelings. The best thing a man can do is to be sensitive and responsive to his wife's fears, her physical and emotional changes, and her needs during her pregnancy, even more so if this is her first. Keep a level head and be prepared for frequent changes in mood, especially toward the end of the pregnancy. Prepare for the unexpected so you can keep things running smoothly and so she can rely on you.

If you still feel frustrated, please remember that men also have their emotional mood swings. So show a little sympathy because you will want the same treatment in return when you have a temper tantrum and vent to her.

When you said "I do" to marriage, you also said "I do" to PMS and mood swings. As I noted earlier, PMS and mood swings don't go away. They will always be a part of your marriage—for better or for worse. You have the power to decide whether you want to make your marriage worse or better. I hope you choose the latter.

— 9 —

Beware the pregnant woman's nesting and spending spree

~ 9 ~

Beware the pregnant woman's nesting and spending spree

During my first wife's first pregnancy, I was not given a heads-up about a pregnant mom's nesting stage. Nor the spending spree associated with it. While I did see and experience the benefits of nesting, I was not privy to the harmful affects of a pregnant mom's out-of-control nesting.

First, let me define nesting and then address the benefits of healthy nesting and the financial hardship it can cause. Nesting is a natural, distinctive urge to prepare for the arrival of the baby. It typically kicks in during the end of the second trimester but can also occur sooner or later depending on the woman. Although nesting is generally associated with pregnant women, nesting is also common with expectant men.

In many cultures, nesting includes activities like naming the baby, selecting and arranging a type of birth, mailing shower invitations, decorating the house and baby's room, attending a baby shower or childbirth class, shopping at the baby accessory store, and assembling furniture. Men nest when they build a room addition, paint the room, or assemble a crib or chair.

These nesting activities can bring a couple closer together for obvious reasons. Mom, dad, and unborn baby are spending time together: time to discuss and make decisions about the decor of the baby's room, style of diaper bag, or name of the baby; to create friendships with other expectant parents; and to organize a support network to take the workload off of you and your wife (see Chapter 14). Any activity related to the preparation of the baby can be considered nesting. And the more you and your wife collaborate in these activities, the stronger your bond with each other will be as a new family.

A mom, however, can take nesting too far. Despite swollen feet, a cumbersome figure, and an aching back, a mom may feel she has to stay busy keeping the house in order, fulfilling obligations that come with being a pregnant mom, or competing with other pregnant moms. All these activities, along with the overscheduling, can physically wear out a mom, which is not good for her or the baby. Instead, a mom needs to conserve her energy for the baby she is carrying and the subsequent birth.

Another danger that results from out-of-control nesting is a compulsive spending spree. This can lead a couple into a financial abyss. But more important, it places more financial pressure on a dad to increase his earning power. So what typically happens is that a man feels that his obligation as a dad is to earn more money working overtime rather than spend more time with his wife and unborn baby.

Compulsive spending can start out small and grow into a destructive habit. It can develop, for example, as a result of low self-esteem brought on by weight gain. The spending then becomes a feel-good drug for the lack of love a mom may feel she is not receiving from her husband, or her insecurities about being a new mom.

Social pressure can also trigger the uncontrollable spending. Your wife may try to improve her status as a mom and turn shopping into a competition with other moms by purchasing the most popular and expensive designer products rather than what she can afford.

There is also immense pressure from advertisers who represent baby accessory stores and companies who sell parenting products. Their aggressive marketing strategy is designed to influence a mom to buy their products. One is the "sale" pitch, which acts like an aphrodisiac and convinces a mom into thinking that if she buys this product, she will save money. No. She won't. You can't save money you spend. If your wife spends $20 on a sale item that originally cost $30, that is still $20 she shouldn't have spent on something she didn't need. In her mind she saved $10, but she really lost $20.

Unfortunately, today's "plastic" culture encourages debt and presents it as a normal, accepted American practice. It is estimated that households with a least one credit card carry an average of about $10,000 in card debt. If at all possible, cut up all the credit cards except one and only use it in case of an emergency.

Look at it this way. Every dollar you and your wife spend means less time spent as a new family. It is important to get a handle on the shopping because overspending can lead to further debt and eventually financial troubles, which ultimately result in stressed relations between a mom and dad. Live within your means and create a realistic budget.

– 10 –

A new dad
can handle finances,
even without any

$\sim 10 \sim$
A new dad can handle finances, even without any

I coined the phrase "The quality of life as a family is more important than the quality of a family's lifestyle." And my wife, Tina, and I have also lived by it.

Not every expectant couple enters parenthood financially stable. Wealth is not a formula for parenting success. Nor is poverty a recipe for failure. I know wealthy parents who have failed in their marriage and relationships with their children. And I know many impoverished parents who have successful marriages and relationships with their children.

To give you a more realistic perspective, let's compare the dynamics of three couples and the real numbers associated with their income and expenses.

Couple #1: Husband is a successful lawyer earning $300,000 per year. His wife is a software engineer earning $120,000 per year. The couple plans to hire a nanny after the birth. They live in an affluent neighborhood, own a home, lease a Mercedes and a Landrover, and are members of a private tennis club. This couple appears to be financially healthy. However, they are not, and, despite their upper-class income, they live beyond their means. Delve into their financial statement and you'll find that they've amassed huge debt. The house mortgage has been refinanced twice. And risky investments added to their financial losses. This couple is living a "borrow-from-Peter-to-pay-Paul" lifestyle.

Couple #2: Husband is a factory worker earning $50,000. Wife works as a waitress earning $30,000. This couple rents an apartment. The husband owns a 1999 Toyota Camry and the wife, a 2001 Honda Civic. Both cars are paid for. The wife plans to quit work and become a stay-at-home mom. This couple lives modestly and has $10,000 in a savings account.

Couple #3: Husband owns a business and earns $50,000 a year. Wife is a schoolteacher earning $80,000. This couple decides to have the husband be the stay-at-home parent. The couple also makes a few unconventional financial decisions. They downsize to a smaller home, which cuts their mortgage payments and property taxes in half. They also move closer to wife's school so she can walk to work and sell one of their two cars.

Yes, there are couples whose finances are in order, but they are few and far between. The majority of couples, many of whom have unplanned pregnancies, don't have theirs in order and struggle to make ends meet. Some couples own homes. Some live in apartments. Some resort to living with their parents. Regardless of financial status or situation, couples will find a way to survive and create the best possible home for their new baby.

If you do the math, you'll discover that many couples overlook the cost associated with the second income. One study showed that the average net gain at the end of the year was about $12,000.

There is also data and research available on the Internet about the "Two-Income Myth." One Web site offers an automatic income calculator, adapted from the book *Shattering the Two-Income Myth* by Andy Dappen. Based on your current personal financial situation, the calculator will show the whole profit and loss analysis of a second income. Another book that explores this myth is *The Two-Income Trap: Why Middle-Class Mothers and Fathers Are Going Broke,* written by Elizabeth Warren and Amelia Warren Tyagi. Here is an excerpt from an interview with Amelia, who discusses a second income.

"The overwhelming majority of us do it because we think it will make our families more secure. But that's not how things have worked out. . . . If you have two people in the workforce, you have double the chance that someone will get laid off, or double the chance that someone could get too sick to work. When that happens, two-income families really get into trouble, and that's how a lot of families quickly go bankrupt."

I'm not suggesting that every couple should become a one-income family. There are plenty of couples that make their two-income family work. What is important is to understand is that whatever your financial situation, there are ways you and your wife can create a budget that will work for your family.

I defer back to that old adage, "It's not about how much you make but rather how much you spend."

Focus on the quality of your life as a family, and you'll be fine.

~ 11 ~

Navigate the medical staff

— 11 —
Navigate the medical staff

One of the biggest cultural shifts in the last twenty years has been the increase in the number of dads who want to be more involved in the pregnancy and birth. The growing number of involved dads is great news. The bad news, however, is that the medical health care industry has ignored or marginalized the need to service new dads.

A major reason is that the educational training medical professionals—receptionists, doctors, childbirth instructors, nurses—receive is only focused on the care and health of moms and babies. Mom and baby are viewed as patients. Dads, on the other hand, are not but should be. And there is significant evidence, as noted in the introduction, to prove that the health care industry has not been attentive and sufficient enough in clinical interactions with the dads.

Therefore, many new dads struggle to navigate their way through a maze of medical professionals who are unprepared to acknowledge them as patients and have no formal educational health care training on how to treat dads or on the subject of fatherhood.

Here are comments from dads who shared their frustrations with me about their experiences with medical professionals.

"The doctor directed all the questions to my wife. He never made eye contact with me. I felt invisible and wondered why I even showed up and took time off of work."

"The childbirth classes aren't very father-friend-ly. All the instructors are women who don't know much about fathering issues. And the curriculum and teaching methods are designed to service the needs of moms and babies."

"I felt like I was treated like a second-class citizen and that my job was to just be a helper for my wife."

"The doctor's lack of attention towards me made me feel like he didn't think my input was important."

"It's a little intimidating to enter an environment where you're not greeted as an equal partner and made to feel like you don't belong there."

As frustrating as it as to deal with a medical system that is not open to changing their behavior in dealing with dads, there are some things you can do to improve the way medical professionals treat you.

First thing you need to buy into is that the medical staff works for you. After all, you and your wife are the customers paying the bill. Granted, you are seeking medical advice from these professionals, but that is what you're paying them for, and as a customer, you should receive the quality service you deserve.

Conducting business with a medical professional is no different than with any other professional, like a realtor. When you hire a realtor to preview houses or a car dealer to buy an automobile, your input is valuable in determining what type of house or car you want to purchase. And you expect quality service and product for your money. The same is true and even more important in the medical industry: you are paying to receive good service and advice.

Establishing a good relationship with the doctor will pay huge dividends throughout the pregnancy, during the birth, and after the birth. The more personal you are, the better service you'll receive. When you're in the office, be respectful, but don't be shy to ask questions. Feel free to also bring a notepad with a list of things you want to discuss, and jot down notes.

If you're not getting what you need from the doctor, don't be afraid to speak up or talk to your wife about finding another doctor.

Next, be a friendly father. Greet the staff with a pleasant smile and handshake. Be aware of your body language. Act like you enjoy being with your wife and that you belong there. Don't behave like you do at the shopping mall while you're waiting for her to finish shopping.

Next, take the initiative to build a friendly relationship with the health professionals (and other expectant moms and dads in classes). People respond more positively and will be more attentive when greeted with a friendly smile and handshake. Help them feel comfortable about having you there. It may take a huge effort on your part to break the ice, but that is okay. In the end, you'll be glad you did.

One tip I offer to new dads is to make at least three visits to the hospital's maternity ward to introduce yourself to the nurses. Choose a morning, early afternoon, and evening time. The point of this exercise is threefold. First is that it will be an opportunity to familiarize yourself with the hospital so that when you bring your wife there, you will know exactly what to do and where everything is. Second, it will be an opportunity to build relationships with the nurses on staff. This way, when you arrive with your wife in labor, the nurses already know who you are and will be more respectful and attentive to your role and needs as a dad. And third, the reason for the different times of the day is that you don't know what time of day your wife will go into labor.

If you feel uncomfortable going alone, invite another expectant dad (or dads) you know or who you have met in the childbirth class. Or invite a male relative or friend.

Your personal touch combined with some fatherly love will benefit not only you but also your wife and new baby. In addition, it will help medical professionals recognize how important and beneficial it will be to make the health system more inclusive and father-friendly.

~ 12 ~

Have a sex talk with the wife

- 12 -
Have a sex talk with the wife

Couples, let alone expectant couples, have a tough time talking about sex in great detail. The word alone instills a feeling of uneasiness. People feel so uncomfortable simply saying the word "sex" that it is easier to have sex than it is to talk about it.

For many men, it is easier to bring up the word "sex" with friends than it is to talk about it with their girlfriend or spouse. And that is because men joke, not talk, about sex. Okay, I can't resist: How often do men like to have sex?

Only on days that start with "T": Tuesday and Thursday, Taturday and Tunday, Today and Tomorrow.

But in a marriage, sex is no joking matter. It is a big deal. And it is even a bigger issue when married couples enter the world of parenthood.

Sex is one of four major topics couples don't talk about enough before and after marriage. (The other three are finances, parenting philosophy, and religion.) I understand that bringing up an intimate, lengthy discussion about sex to your wife is not easy. But the more a person ignores the subject, the more uncomfortable it is to have a conversation about it.

Remember, sex, and the intimacy and romance that comes with it, is what brought you and your wife closer together and into wedlock. After wedlock sex is necessary in nurturing and strengthening the bond in your marriage. Marriage without sex is a lonely feeling and can tear a couple apart.

There is a legitimate reason couples never establish a habit of discussing sex. During the teenage years, sex education took a "birds-and-the-bees" approach that involved fear-mongering tactics. Sex was also presented more as a dirty or bad act. Any serious conversation about the pros and benefits of sex was never brought up. The good news is that it is not too late to start talking about sex and renew a positive attitude about it!

So how do you begin?

Well, either you or your wife has to break the ice. If you wait for her, the conversation may never come up. This was the case in my marriage. So I made the first move. I figured I had nothing to lose and a lot to gain. My conversations with Tina led me to come up with the following list that compares the different ways men and women think about and view sex before and during pregnancy. I think this brief list will help you feel more comfortable discussing sex with your wife.

What a woman may not know about how a man really feels about sex

A man thinks about sex more often, has no control over his sex drive or blood flow to his penis (just as a woman has not control over her PMS), and can have as many as two or three spontaneous erections a day. When a man does not have sex, he suffers from MSB—Multiple Sperm Backup. Sex is good exercise and more physical than emotional. Still, the word "sex" is synonymous with intimacy. Sex is the language of intimacy and is how a man expresses his feelings about a woman. A man is visual and more interested in the deed. Sex is also a stress reliever; the time a husband spends having sex with his wife is an escape from reality.

What a woman (or man) may not know about a man's feelings about sex after pregnancy

Not every husband is turned on by his wife's pregnancy. An expectant dad's sex drive may diminish because he fears he may hurt the baby. He may be turned off by a growing abdomen, leaking breasts, or symptoms of pregnancy his wife is experiencing, like nausea (hardly an aphrodisiac). He may feel awkward because it feels like someone else is in the room, especially if he knows the baby is a girl. And yes, a husband may be aroused by his pregnant wife's new physique.

What a man may not know about how a woman really feels about sex

The environment influences a woman's sex drive, and the ceremony of sex is more important than the deed. Sex is work and more emotional than physical. The word sex is not synonymous with intimacy. A woman's sexual desire originates between her ears, not between her legs.

What a man (or woman) may not know about sex during the pregnancy

During pregnancy, a woman suffers from PMS, and her mood swings increase. Her body, especially her breasts, may become more sensitive to touch. She may struggle with self-esteem and feel unattractive due to weight gain. Fatigue may make it difficult for her to find the energy to have sex. She may feel that a mother isn't supposed to have sex and also fear hurting the baby. And, yes, a wife's sex drive can also increase during pregnancy.

The challenging issues a couple may run into is that only one of the spouse's sex drive stays the same or increases while the other has no interest in sex. Or a couple's timing may be off. A dad may be in the mood but the wife may not, and vice versa.

Then there is the issue of a pregnant woman not having the ability to engage in sex for health reasons. In this case, a husband may need to resort to short-term celibacy, which a man has experienced before during his single years.

Regardless of a couple's situation, the sex issue is resolvable through a greater understanding of each other's feelings and needs through good communication. No matter how uncomfortable a new mom and dad may be, it is important to honestly discuss how each of them really feels about sex.

~ 13 ~

Guess what? A new dad is not alone

– 13 –
Guess what? A new dad is not alone

Whenever a new dad enters my expectant dads' class (for dads only), he aimlessly strolls in with the same kind of apprehension he did when he accompanied his pregnant wife to the Lamaze class or a clothing store. I see it in the body language and expression on his face. He'd rather be somewhere else, like the golf course, a sporting event, a bar, the gym—anywhere but with a room full of dads he hardly knows to discuss how they feel about becoming fathers.

After brief introductions, the dads begin to feel comfortable about the setting and recognize that this is not the touchy-feely, lecture-based session they had anticipated. I ask the dads why they have come to the class.

Most answer, "My wife made me."

A few answer, "To learn how to be a better dad."

Next, I ask the dads to share one concern they have about being a dad.

Most of the dads struggle to admit they have any issues. Some dads are clueless and acknowledge that they came to find out what they should be concerned about. Generally, only five of the twenty-five dads find the courage to give an honest answer, and the rest ditto the concerns.

As I write a list of additional issues on the white board, the dads discover that there are more issues they hadn't considered or have overlooked, issues that include mom's and baby's health, his mortality (dying and leaving his child fatherless), paternity (is the child really mine?), performance in the delivery room, fear of the unknown, finances, lifestyle change, bonding, sex, managing the household, balancing a new schedule, pets, handling advice, dealing with grandparents, asking for help, and building a support team.

"After seeing the list, I never considered asking for help and building a support team as issues," one participant commented.

The mood in the class suddenly changes. The anxiety diminishes, and interest in learning more about the issues written on the board increases with each dad who speaks up. One dad after another piggybacks off of an issue mentioned by another dad that leads to a discussion about another fathering issue. The dads are so engaged in conversation that they forget that two hours have passed.

Before the class ends, I ask the dads to share one thing they have learned that day.

The most common answer? "I learned that I'm not alone and that other men feel the same way I do about being a new dad. I'm so glad that my wife made me attend this class. I'm going to thank her when I get home."

So why do men feel alone and emotionally isolated? The answer lies in how our culture has raised boys. Boys are taught not to share their concerns and feelings. To do so would result in being labeled a "pansy," "sissy," or "gay." The message is clear: suck it up and take it like a man. Then by the time a boy reaches manhood, he is hesitant to admit and address his fears and insecurities.

After the announcement of the pregnancy, there are many emotions running through a new dad's mind. The initial reaction is shock, followed by pride and excitement, then anxiety and concerns about his future role as a dad. A new dad can experience the same high and low mood swings as a mom. Sadly, a new dad's natural response is to clam up, because to admit fears and concerns is a sign of weakness. Eventually, he masters the art of masking his emotions and wanders aimlessly into the world of fatherhood. Therefore, it is no surprise that a new dad is under the impression he is a lone wolf with nowhere to reach out for help or support.

What did surprise me at first was the relief on the faces and in the voices of the dads after they heard the other dads in the room had similar emotions and concerns. Another surprise was how comfortable the diverse group of dads felt about sharing their concerns with a room full of other dads they just met. One dad told me that he had never talked to his wife about a couple of the concerns brought up in class.

"I have never been asked to share how I really felt or been given permission to voice a concern I have. It felt good to get it off my chest."

"I appreciate being able to share how I feel without being judged or criticized. Another thing I liked is that no one questioned my masculinity and that what I'm feeling is normal."

"I know I didn't say much during the discussions but I learned a lot from listening to all of you. It's nice to know that other dads struggle with the same issues I was afraid to address."

"I feel so relieved and look forward to sharing what I've learned from you guys today with my wife."

I've been conducting workshops for dads since 1992. Trust me. You're not alone.

— 14 —

Ask for help and build a support network for your family

– 14 –

Ask for help and build a support network for your family

Why does it take a million sperm to fertilize one egg?

Because the male sperm will not ask for directions.

A sking for help is not one of a man's strongest traits because of the cowboy mentality I touched on in the previous chapter.

Seeking help and support are not signs of weakness. In fact, you should view it as a sign of courage and strength. To not accept help to establish a support team is not a wise decision because it will place you, your wife, and your baby's physical health in jeopardy. And not having help available will also increase the stress level during and after the pregnancy, especially if your wife becomes bedridden.

I understand most people, especially men, struggle to ask for help. A little has to do with the fear of surrendering control and feeling indebted. But I'm not going to discuss in great detail the psychology of why because the bottom line is that you need to ask for help and accept it. I'm here to tell you it's okay to get help and to give you permission to do so whenever you need it. Quite often men ask for help or support *after* a crisis. Don't wait for one to happen. A new dad must be proactive and take preventative measures to increase his chances of protecting his family from any imminent danger when it may occur. I'll elaborate on a new dad's role as the protector in Chapter 18.

In Chapter 11, I offered suggestions on how to encourage the medical staff to acknowledge you as a dad and properly service the needs of you, your wife, and your baby. Now I'm going to do the same by encouraging you to gain help from your relatives, friends, neighbors, coworkers, and others who should be a part of your home support team. Here are some steadfast rules to make you more comfortable when it comes to getting the help you need.

Asking for help can be delivered from a position of strength. After you ask, you're the one who will delegate the chores and have control. Divide and conquer. Don't outsource the chores to just three or four people; find as many people as you can. This way, if one of your support staff becomes ill, you will have another person to fill the spot.

If the help will improve your situation, then you should ask, and if your request is within reason, people will likely say yes. People want to help, but they can't if you don't let them know you want help or what you need. If a person willingly offers or gives help, it is not charity.

If you don't ask, you won't get.

There are two ways asking for help can be accomplished. The first is to be direct and initiate the request. "Tina and I need help. I'm organizing a support team for my new family. Would you like to be a part of that team?" If he answers yes, then follow up with, "Here is a list of ways you can help. Which one would you like to choose?"

The second way is when another person asks you one of the following two questions: "How are you and your wife doing?" or "Do you need any help?"

The immediate and natural response to the first question is always, "Everything is good," or "Okay." The second automatic response is "No." In either case, you are not being truthful. Life is not always okay or good. Everyone has ups and downs, and we all need a little help to smooth out whatever little bump in the road comes our way. No matter how much you think you don't need help, there is at least one task or job another person can help you with to make your life a little easier. Look at it this way. Each task a person does for you means one less thing you need to do, which serves two purposes. One is it that it will relieve stress. Two is that it will give you more time to spend and enjoy with your new family.

After a person commits to helping, give her the list that can include cleaning chores, cooking pre-cooked meals, washing the car, mowing the lawn, doing the grocery shopping, house repairs, laundry, assembling furniture, or running errands. Here are a few specific examples of favors to include.

One request can be to have a person paint the baby's room. Mom can give her input on the colors and design, but let someone else paint the room for obvious reasons.

One person can be responsible for cleaning the house while you and your wife are giving birth to the baby at the hospital. This way you come home to a clean house—and one less thing to worry about.

Another person can be responsible for mailing the birth announcements and thank you cards. Your wife can sign the thank you cards, and the helper can address the envelopes then stamp and mail them.

Employers and coworkers can also be a great source of help at work. Ask some of your coworkers to temporarily take on a portion of your workload.

The more people involved, the less each person has to do to cover for you. The extra time you have can be used for doctor's appointments with your wife.

Building a support team for your new family is necessary during the pregnancy and even more important after the baby's birth. By that time you'll have an efficient running support team to help with the additional work needed to care for a baby. Trust me, there will be a lot more work ahead of you.

If all the work involved in building a support team sounds a bit overwhelming, let me remind you that as the dad, you have the easy part.

— 15 —

Being a new dad will affect friendships

– 15 –

Being a new dad will affect friendships

After the wedding my lifestyle and priorities changed because I had another person in my life to care for and think about: Tina. As husband and wife, Tina and I had to check in with each other before making decisions or replying to invitations from friends. Many of my single male friends had a hard time understanding why I had to consult Tina before giving them an answer. As you can imagine, the conversation quickly turned into a busting-my-chops session that included name-calling and questioning my masculinity. Even some of my married male friends, who lived by a stepford-wife code, laid into me with "Hey, Hogan, who wears the pants in the family?"

After Tina and I announced her pregnancy, my life and priorities changed again. This time, the changes were more dramatic and the stress level a little higher. The new baby meant making a greater commitment, and giving up a little more independence and freedom. Which also meant I had to alter my social life and the nature of my friendships. And being the social butterfly that I am, the adjustment was very difficult.

There is no question that becoming a new dad will affect your relationship with your single and married-without-children male friends. Spontaneous rendezvous like last-minute trips to Las Vegas or a bite to eat after a day at the office is out of the question. You'll also have fewer nights available to go out with your friends. They may stop calling because they think you're neglecting them or are too busy (which you are) or aren't interested in having a good time with them anymore. You may also feel like you have less in common and temporarily stop calling them.

I understand that an invitation to a sporting event like an NBA, NFL, or MLB game, fishing or hunting trip, round of golf, or drinks at the sports bar after a day at the office is tough to turn down and much more appealing than hanging out with a pregnant wife at home. But the bottom line is that your priorities must change. Your pregnant wife and unborn baby's needs come before any friend, and it's your responsibility to convey that message to your friends.

If a friend doesn't accept and understand your situation, then maybe he isn't worth having as a friend. And that is okay. Is he really the kind of friend you can count on or want to have around, especially during this crucial time in your life as a new dad? Is he the kind of friend you want your child to eventually meet and hang out with?

A friend is easy to dump. A wife and baby are not. Good friends don't let their friend abandon his new family. However, if your friend is supportive, here are some suggestions to strengthen and keep your friendship alive. Remind him that there is great value in these activities for both you and him because he may become a dad someday.

1. Invite him to accompany you to visit the nurse in the maternity ward at the hospital.
2. Invite him to accompany you to an expectant dad's class.
3. Invite him to carry out one of the tasks on your support team list (see Chapter 13).
4. Invite him to the baby shower.
5. Invite him to shop with you at the baby accessory store. Get breakfast before or after you shop.

Although you may lose a few friends, you'll have plenty of opportunities to establish new male friendships. You'll meet plenty of other expectant dads in the childbirth classes and connect with other dads in your neighborhood.

One of my favorite adages is "The choice you make makes you." Your choice of friends also makes you. As you build your support network, choose and keep friends who will bring out the best in you as a husband and new dad and who you can count on. The true friends are the ones who will be there for you when you, your wife, and your unborn baby need them the most.

– 16 –

Define your own role as a dad

– 16 –

Define your own role as a dad

In the 1960s men were given clear-cut roles that defined their masculinity as husbands and dads. Dad was a shadowy figure who left home at dawn and returned at dusk. His role was measured by how hard he worked and how much he earned. After work dad was the visible disciplinarian who didn't talk much, ask for help, or show any emotion. He was a macho man who never showed any sign of weakness nor helped out with the household chores.

During the 1970s and 1980s, the feminist movement liberated women to expand their professional careers and roles as mothers and also attacked traditional male roles and beliefs. Men became so confused as to how they should behave that it inspired author Bruce Feirstein to write a tongue-and-cheek book, *Real Men Don't Eat Quiche,* satirizing stereotypes of masculinity. A year later in 1983, the movie *Mr. Mom* was released. Although this movie and Feirstein's book poked fun at the raging battle between the sexes, they had a telling effect on American men and forced them to question and reexamine their traditional roles.

Ironically, as the feminist movement marched on with more career opportunities opening up for women, it liberated men to explore and participate in parenting duties that were once reserved only for women. As a result, the role men played in parenting changed dramatically.

Seven years after *Mr. Mom*'s release, the increasing number of successful women in the workplace ignited an at-home-dads revolution. The at-home dads proved that men were just as capable as women in nurturing, caring for, and raising a child, but more important, that trading a tool belt for an apron didn't mean a dad lost his masculinity.

At-home dads served as a wake-up call to fatherhood just as the feminist did to corporate America. Now, "real men not only eat quiche but also bake it."

As our society grew to accept and appreciate at-home dads, another alternative lifestyle for dads emerged: flextime. Flextime is any work arrangement that is not a traditional eight-to-five job. This includes both full-time and part-time positions, project work, freelance, shift work, weekends, and a compressed workweek. The professions include factory workers, janitors, policemen, musicians, waiters, firefighters, medical professionals, and attorneys. Many employers offer four ten-hour-day workweeks or let their employees work from home.

Although not every man has the ability or desire to be an at-home dad, flextime offers the traditional working man an opportunity to still be a breadwinner and also spend time with his children. The intent of flextime parenting is to have one parent at home while the other is at work, which means that a dad has to accept shared responsibility in the domestic duties and day-to-day care of the baby.

Due to work flexibility, in the past couple of decades, traditional working men have voluntarily and intentionally been placing their careers on hold or changing their work schedules to be available as hands-on caregivers for their children. These unconventional choices flextime dads made were totally out of character but welcomed with open arms.

The at-home and flextime-dad phenomenon definitely influenced more men to change their attitude about fatherhood for the better. The result has been happier, healthier, enthusiastic dads who have become more comfortable showing off their nurturing side—in a masculine way, of course!

Consider yourself lucky. Today is a good time to be a dad because there is a broader definition and acceptance of what a dad can do and be. A dad now has three options instead of one: working, using flextime, or being an at-home dad. With your wife, decide which will work best for your new family.

You now have a sense of empowerment that most dads didn't have before and can define your own role as a dad.

― 17 ―

Speak up—let a dad's voice be heard

— 17 —

Speak up—let a dad's voice be heard

I wish I could honestly tell you that the parenting world is father-friendly. But it's not. The bad news is that an expectant dad is not viewed and treated as an equal partner. This is evident by the childbirth instructor's use of the word "coach" and huge imbalance among education, resource, and support services available for moms versus dads. The good news is that you can change this social problem by being proactive and speaking up.

I understand that for legitimate reasons, you may be gun-shy about speaking up. It may not be in your nature. If you are an introvert, you'll be less likely to speak your mind because you may feel insecure and intimidated about offering an opinion. You may not feel it is your place to offer your opinion and don't want to be accused of being an overbearing trouble-maker. If I may be blunt: whatever the reason, get over it. There is too much at stake. What if you don't speak up? Later down the road you may find yourself wishing you did.

Another major reason to speak up is to make yourself visible and let people know that you are an equal partner in the parenting venture. You must speak up to develop your identity and value as a dad, or else they will assume that you are not interested and continue treating you as an invisible person.

Before you speak up, there is one important thing you need to know: view each unfriendly father moment you experience as a teachable moment. When you do speak up, your tone of voice and the way you deliver your message will be vital in obtaining the positive results you want to achieve. First, however, let me give you a better understanding of why our society is not as father-friendly as it should be.

"Family-friendly" doesn't necessarily mean "father-friendly." Although the medical and health industry, companies, schools, churches, and organizations profess to be family-and-father-friendly, most have only provided lip service. I can support this claim by simply counting the number of support services available for moms in comparison to those for dads, and likewise with the amount of funding. As I noted in Chapter 11, the medical health care industry doesn't provide much guidance and assistance to their employees on how to properly service dads. What complicates matters is that most of the employees are women. A female-dominated staff makes it next to impossible for the childbirth instructors there to empathize with and know how to service the needs of dads. Another major factor is the liability issue. A hospital must follow government regulations that include a list of legal requirements that have to be met, most of which pertain to servicing the needs of the mom and baby and providing classes for them. That translates into very little time or commitment to provide classes for and about dads.

Another example is the childbirth instructor's failure to acknowledge the pregnant wife's husband as "dad." After I attended several childbirth classes, I was frustrated with the instructor's constant reference to me as coach, partner, or significant other. I asked the instructor why she didn't just refer to me as a dad. She said, "We are being sensitive to the couples who aren't married." I explained to her how insulted I felt and then asked her why it was okay to be insensitive to a man like me who demonstrated his commitment to his wife and baby through marriage. I was so excited about being a new dad, and now my title was being taken from me, and I no longer felt like an equal partner. Twenty-two years later, despite that the majority of couples are married, childbirth instructors continue in the best interest of political correctness to use the terms "coach," "partner," and "significant other." Sometimes what you say may fall on deaf ears, but that's okay, because what's important is that you speak up.

The medical staff is also not properly trained in how to make the hospital environment father-friendly. Even the best intentions by medical professionals usually reap negative results. For example, Pat, a childbirth instructor, was proud to point out how she made the waiting room father-friendly with one poster of a dad cradling a newborn. Next to that poster was another poster with a sultry photo of an eighteen-year-old girl with a message about preventing teenage pregnancy. "Pat," I told her, "there is no way a dad will even notice the poster with the dad. His eyes will be fixed on the other poster. And then his wife will slap him for having a wandering eye." She replied, "Wow, Hogan, I never even thought of that." She then took the poster of the girl down.

The lack of attention given to a dad that can lead him to feel ignored, marginalized, and alienated also exists in his place of work, home, and community.

Although some companies offer their male employees paternity leave under the Family Medical Leave Act as well as other provisions, they aren't necessarily sincere in providing these services for dads. And a dad may not feel comfortable using any of the provisions. In fact, research shows that most dads don't take advantage of them due to fear of jeopardizing a promotion or their jobs. Although the concept of a dad's loyalty to family before work doesn't fly with most employers, it doesn't mean you shouldn't utilize the company's services.

If you do speak up and are not happy with your employer's reaction, policies, or views regarding your desire to be a more involved father, you do have another option or two: explore the idea of looking to work for another company that is father-friendly, or change professions. Yes, this is a huge risk; however, it may be a choice available to you. But first discuss it with your wife.

In your home and community you will also experience a lack of respect for the significant role you play as a new dad. You'll receive backhanded comments and opinions you don't agree with from your wife, relatives, friends, and strangers.

Here are some stories from expectant dads who graduated from one of my classes, where they learned the technique of how to speak up. Their stories will best describe the benefits of speaking up.

"Prior to the birth, my wife, the doctor, and I agreed that I would cut the umbilical cord. I explained how important it was for me to do the procedure and my way of expressing my personal daddy-bond with our baby. After the birth, the doctor grabbed the sterile scissors and proceeded to cut the umbilical cord. That split second I decided to speak up. I reminded the doctor of our agreement. The doctor apologized and stated that she was so used to cutting it that she had forgotten. She handed the sterile scissors to me. I was so glad I spoke up."

"My wife kept insisting that she wanted her mom in the delivery room. I didn't want to share this special intimate moment with my mother-in-law or anyone else except my wife. . . . I asked my wife why

her mom's feelings were more important than mine. I also told her that this is our family, not [her] mom's. . . . My wife apologized and honored my request."

"The medical assistant from the OB-GYN called. She called to ask for some more personal information and share some news from the doctor about the unborn baby. I told her that my wife was sleeping. The medical assistant asked if my wife could call her back. I told her that I'm the dad and that she can ask me the questions and share the doctor's information with me."

"I got tired of having the childbirth instructor calling me coach and partner. I was the dedicated husband and dad. I spoke to her after the class, told her how I felt, and asked her if she would please refer to me as the 'dad.' She didn't, but I felt good because at least I spoke up."

"After I read two books about pregnancy, my wife asked me to read another book. I asked her why I have to keep reading books about a pregnant mom and unborn baby but she didn't about what I'm going through as a father. She apologized and asked me to buy her a fatherhood book she could read."

What I hope you learn from these stories is that just because the environment is not father-friendly doesn't mean you can't evoke change for yourself and eventually for other dads. The reality is that a dad has his own unique questions, concerns, and needs. They should be addressed because your comments and opinions matter. So speak up.

— 18 —

Establish a protective boundary for *your* new family

– 18 –

Establish a protective boundary for *your* new family

The need for a man to protect a person he loves from harm is instinctive. Being a protector is one of three core principles in which a man measures his masculinity, the other two being provider and disciplinarian.

Most men view their role as protector in the physical sense, and more often than not, they take action only after a threat occurs. If a person, especially a stranger, spoke in anger or acted disrespectfully to your wife, that person's action would trigger you to stand up in her defense.

There is also another aspect to being a protector that most men often fail to understand and recognize. Protection is not just a reactive behavior. It can also be a proactive one in which a dad avoids a potential threat to someone he cares for—in this case, the mom, baby, and you. Making sure you and your wife wear a seat belt is a proactive gesture to minimize the injuries all of you could suffer if an accident occurred. Opening up a savings account to save money for a rainy day protects your family from any financial hardship.

Being proactive is also great way to maximize your role as protector and give you more value as a dad. A new dad can be proactive in setting boundaries to protect his new family from overbearing relatives, friends, and neighbors. But putting this into practice is a whole other ball game because these are relatives and people within your social circle who you will depend on for support. So it will require you and your wife to exercise great discipline in establishing a united front and making some minor adjustments to your lifestyle. Pregnancy and parenthood are difficult enough without people invading a new pregnant couple's personal space. This is a time when you and your wife need each other's undivided attention. Overbearing people with their unrealistic demands, intrusions, and unannounced visits can disrupt the flow of your life as new parents.

News of a wife's pregnancy spreads like wildfire, and everyone in your social circle, especially the women, will want to involve themselves in your new life as a family. Although these people have good intentions and their involvement can be useful, it can become overbearing and cause friction in your marriage. Therefore, you and your wife should establish a boundary with a set of rules to ensure people will not invade the personal space designated for your new family.

Begin with a short list and add on when necessary. Don't overwhelm yourself and others with a long list of regulations; the rules aren't as important as enforcing them. Whatever the rules are, make sure you set limits, define what is and isn't allowed, and offer opportunities for people to be involved without invading your personal space. If you present the boundaries and rules in a united front, you shouldn't have any problems with people breaking them. However, in case someone does, have a set of agreed-upon consequences.

The most common people who overstep their boundaries are mothers and mothers-in-law. They of all people will be the most difficult to deal with. In either case, make sure both of you approach her face-to-face. If it is your mother, you do the talking. If it is your mother-in-law, your wife should speak. Both of you may find this confrontation difficult. It's natural for a wife and husband to fear their moms, especially when they fear losing their inheritance. Nevertheless, it is important to overcome this fear as soon as possible. Remind your mother (or have your wife remind your mother-in-law) that this is your family, not hers. When you talk with her, be specific about how you feel and give her an option.

"Mom we're having a tough time adjusting to the pregnancy and all the wonderful people offering to help. To manage our life a little better, Karen and I have created a list and calendar of how people can help. If you really want to help, Tuesday is a good day for you to help with the laundry and maybe have lunch with Karen."

"My mom kept pressuring us with names for our unborn baby. We finally sat down with her and asked her to stop lobbying for her choice of names."

And if a pow-wow with mother or mother-in-law doesn't work, use the third-party rule I noted in Chapter 7.

"My mother was spending way too much time at our house. I asked my brother to talk to my mom. He pointed out to her how many times she'd been to our house and kindly suggested that she back off. It worked."

Brothers, sisters, friends, and neighbors will be easier to deal with. However, there are some preventative measures you can take to diffuse overbearing people. Talk to the most trusted person you feel comfortable with in your family and share your intentions. Support from him or her will validate and give credibility to your game plan.

Make copies of a calendar with specific times you want privacy, and create a "to-do" list to hand out to people. This way people know the agenda and who does what. It will also give an opportunity for people to trade days or chores.

Train yourself to not be so quick to answer the phone or the doorbell. By not answering the phone, you and your wife have control of the boundary. Instead, on your answering machine give a brief message such as: "Hello, thanks for calling. We're adjusting to our busy life as new parents. We appreciate the phone call and will get back to you as soon as we have time available." This is also a useful tip after the birth of the baby, when people call to make sure everyone is okay and to know the baby's name, date of birth, health, weight, and height. Add this information to the answering machine.

The purpose of these exercises is to prevent unannounced visits and interruptions. You, your wife, and your baby will need quiet time to bond as a new family, which can't happen with constant disruptions.

People will treat you the way you train them: if you give them an inch, you'll become a human doormat. Once they invade your personal space, it will be much harder to persuade them to withdraw and follow rules.

The wonderful thing about establishing a boundary is that people will respect it as long as you and your wife hold your ground. Be straightforward and let people know what is and is not acceptable. Initially, a few people may express their disapproval, but that's okay. Let them vent, but stand your ground.

~ 19 ~

Anxiety about the delivery room is normal

− 19 −

Anxiety about the delivery room is normal

E ven though a new dad looks forward to this memorable moment that will bring great joy into his life, he also carries a great deal of concern about what will happen in the delivery room. For so many new dads, it is the video in the childbirth classes that induces the anxiety.

The video paints an unflattering picture of what occurs in the delivery room. A lot of attention is placed on the chaos, sweat, and gruesome pain a mom endures before and during the delivery. I have never understood why the instructors show the video because it seems that the bleak images only exacerbate the anxiety a new dad feels. Concerns about the delivery room are valid, but there is no reason to lose sleep over it. Here's one testimonial about a father's delivery room anxiety: "In the expectant dad class I attended, one of the veteran dads, who brought his baby, admitted and shared his anxiety and how he overcame it. He gave me great comfort in knowing that I wasn't alone and that I would survive."

A new dad's anxiety can range from feeling squeamish about fainting to being concerned about his wife's and baby's health. Even for the most machismo man, the mere sight of blood and fluids can cause him to faint. Fainting and having a nurse haul you off in a wheelchair while you're wearing an oxygen mask can be humiliating. The fear of fainting also evokes a dad to worry about being a distraction or hindrance, which can jeopardize his wife and baby's health. But don't worry about the medical staff. They've done this procedure thousands of times. However, if something doesn't look or feel right to you, ask. (Remember the umbilical cord story in Chapter 17.)

Other concerns include bumping and knocking over an important piece of equipment, or seeing your wife in pain, especially during a C-section. For most new dads, it's a horrible sight to see a doctor stick a knife in his wife's belly.

A new dad may also worry about the health and condition of the baby. Will the baby have a deformity or be missing a limb? Will the baby be born with a rare genetic disease? Will the baby be born disabled? I'll elaborate on this topic in Chapter 25.

Another anxiety stems from a new dad being unsure of the nature and purpose of his presence. You may be uncertain about your role and job title: Are you the coach, cheerleader, spectator, director, photographer, or cameraman?

Whatever your perception is about the delivery room, nothing can adequately prepare you for the real thing, so why worry over situations you can't control? What you can control is how mentally prepared you will be to react if something does go wrong in the delivery room. As I've discussed, take a proactive approach to minimize the number of concerns that bother you. Write a list of your concerns on paper. Acknowledge them, stop fretting about the ones you cannot control, and mentally prepare yourself to address them if they happen. Recognize the anxiety, but don't fret about it because if you do, it will distract you from enjoying the birth.

Approach your anxiety the way a fireman, doctor, or nurse prepares for their profession. A fireman knows the dangers of entering a burning building. He has anxieties about his job, but he has mentally and physically prepared himself to deal with the fears because the end result of saving a person is the ultimate goal. The same is true with doctors and nurses. Their job is to keep your wife and baby alive and well.

As a new dad, focus on your goal, which is to enjoy the experience and welcome the baby. It is the doctors' and nurses' goal and job to care for your wife and baby and maintain the equipment. You can't control the health of your wife and baby or what might happen to you. Stop worrying about fainting. Relinquish your anxieties to the doctor and nurses because they are trained to handle any situations that may arise. Have faith in the people you hire.

There is, however, one anxiety you can control. If you are confused about your role, don't be. You have only one: to be a dad. The most common mistake a new dad makes is that he forgets to be a dad.

In my first birth I was so worried about directing traffic, photographing and videoing, and comforting my wife that I spent most of my time playing the role of director, producer, photographer, and unregistered nurse and forgot to act like a dad.

Witnessing a birth is indescribable. It is one of those "you-have-to-be-there" moments in life that you can only experience for yourself. If you focus too much on your anxiety, you won't be able do your job and enjoy the birth of the baby as a dad.

– 20 –

Nurture the marriage

– 20 –

Nurture the marriage

Once you and your wife announce the pregnancy, the dynamics of the husband-wife relationship change dramatically. The titles of "mom" and "dad" put a whole new twist on the marriage. Look at how much your relationship changed when the two of you went from boyfriend and girlfriend to husband and wife. The change was for the better, but with it came a few adjustments that tested the strength of your relationship. This also applies to the transition of being a childless married couple to becoming expectant parents.

During the pregnancy, the unborn baby and mom are the main focus of attention, the costars of the show. Dad, unfortunately and unintentionally, lives in the shadow of the baby and mom—which you are probably already experiencing as you read this book.

While the unborn baby will bring great joy, life becomes more challenging and complicated because there is a third person in the mix. As a new dad, you'll be competing for attention with the unborn baby. A mom's natural instinct is to focus all of her attention on the unborn baby first, herself second, and the husband third. This means you will no longer be your wife's main squeeze. It doesn't mean she doesn't love you, but her actions and non-actions will give you that impression. The end result is that a new dad will feel neglected. If a dad doesn't address this very serious issue during the pregnancy, it will escalate to the tenth degree or higher after the baby is born, when instead of having to split your time between two people, you'll be splitting it with three. The pressure increases to find time to nurture your marriage, but it has to be done.

The most important thing you need to know is that your wife will probably not recognize the harm in placing the mother-child relationship before the husband-wife relationship. Therefore, it is up to you to bring it to her attention and help her understand that your marriage comes before the baby.

In your wife's defense, our culture has indoctrinated this notion that mom's first priority is to the baby. I contend that it's not, and the increasing divorce rate supports my conclusion. Spousal neglect plays a large part in couples filing for divorce.

Let me use the airplane oxygen mask analogy to prove my point. What is the first thing the stewardess instructs couples with children to do if the oxygen levels in the main cabin become unstable? That when the oxygen masks drop down, place your mask on first and then secure your child's. Why? There is the risk that you may pass out before you are even able to put the mask on your child. This same risk applies to a marriage. If you and your wife don't give attention (oxygen) to each other first, the marriage won't survive. If the marriage doesn't survive, there will be no family.

So how do you supply oxygen to your marriage? You nurture the friendship part of your marriage with affection and acts of kindness. (Sex is not a part of the nurturing process.) Now, you may be thinking, Why do I have to take the initiative? Why can't my wife just give me the attention I need? Remember Chapter 6? If your EGO is still here, get rid of it. Remember Chapter 17? You need to be proactive and speak up (not hide in your man cave) to prevent your marriage from going stale and possibly failing. Don't wait for your marriage to break apart piece by piece and then try to repair it.

If you come across a stumbling block with your wife, communicate to her how you feel. Let her know you feel ignored. She may not be aware. Remind her and give her suggestions as to how she can help nurture the marriage; she can't read your mind. And refrain from passive-aggressive behavior that will only make the situation worse. Good communication is essential in nurturing and maintaining a happy marriage.

Your first course of action is to schedule a regular date night with your wife. I suggest at least once a month, but twice a month is better. There is, however, one rule: no discussions about the unborn baby. This is a lot easier said than done. If one of you has a slip of the tongue and mentions the unborn baby, acknowledge it and then change the subject. You may want to post your regular date night on the calendar that I suggested you hand out to your support team. Hey, someone may give you free movie tickets or a gift card for a dinner at a local restaurant, thereby saving you money.

Let me clarify what I mean by a date. A date doesn't have to involve spending a great deal of money. After all, your budget changes with another mouth to feed and support. A date can be an hour walk in the park or on the beach, pizza and a beverage at a local pizza parlor, a visit to the museum, making popcorn and watching a movie at home, attending a free community concert and bringing your own food, or going to an amusement park and taking a picture together in the photo booth.

A quick side note: don't drop the dating ball after the baby is born. Don't allow the new baby to interfere with your marriage. There will be plenty of people available to help care for the baby.

To help you plan out an activity, write a list of activities or places you visited before your marriage and the pregnancy. It should be a long list. From that list, choose one for your next date. Talk about the memories you have of that place, and make new ones.

The point of dating while your wife is pregnant is to take a break from the pregnancy and life's challenges, and to have fun being a married couple!

~ 21 ~

Embrace fatherhood

— 21 —
Embrace fatherhood

Honey, I'm pregnant!" Tina exclaimed. "Really? All right," I replied. Then I hugged her.

For the next eight months, Tina's jubilation intensified each time she greeted someone with news of the pregnancy. She was proud to be a mom and embraced motherhood with a passion that had been building up in her since she was a little girl.

I, on the other hand, had mixed emotions. I went from shock to reality to panic to having reservations about being a father. All kinds of fears ran through my mind. I didn't embrace fatherhood in the same way Tina did motherhood. When I was a boy, my list of what I wanted to be when I grew up included pro athlete, policeman, fireman, or entrepreneur. Fatherhood was the last thing on my mind.

While Tina was looking forward to her new life as a mother, I was running scared and questioning my decision to be a dad. I began to think about how this baby was going to alter and possibly ruin a lifestyle I was accustomed to living. The more I thought about being a dad, the longer my list of concerns grew. Eventually, the worrisome list overshadowed what little joy I felt in being a dad and discouraged any desire I had left to embrace fatherhood.

Why don't most men embrace fatherhood with the same exuberance most women do in embracing motherhood? Unplanned pregnancies notwithstanding, most men refrain from depositing the emotional investment necessary to begin and sustain a relationship with another human being for various cultural and personal reasons, some of which have been addressed. Based on my life, I believe the major reason is that most men know how to measure self-worth only by tangible assets.

For example, the compensation and reward for investing in work is a paycheck, an award like a plaque or a car. When a man invests in a sport, it is the winning score or wager on a bet. When he invests in a contest, there is a trophy or prize money. Tangible payment and instant gratification is not the result of a man investing his time and work into a relationship with an unborn baby.

Granted, after the birth, the baby is tangible, but the depth and quality of a father-child relationship is immeasurable. As they say, spending time with a child is priceless. An unborn baby is also not capable of giving any instant feedback that translates into a tangible asset, so there is no instant gratification with the relationship.

Okay, so you're a new dad. You're already struggling to manage a relationship with your spouse, and now you're being asked to invest more of yourself and time (that you feel you don't have) into an unborn baby. You feel overwhelmed and concerned about how you will find the time. The key is to make time to embrace fatherhood. It's not that you aren't capable. You are!

I understand that the cards may be stacked against you to succeed as a new dad, but you have choices. One is to wallow in self-pity. You can choose to remain emotionally distant and make a long list of excuses to justify your behavior, which is the easy thing to do and the route most men take. And regardless of whatever hurtful past a new dad has experienced, he has the power to change his behavior and attitude for the better. You can't edit the past, but you can change the future.

Another choice is to embrace fatherhood and reap the rewards of the investment you put into being a new dad. You can stop making excuses and focus on what will give you a deeper emotional connection to your unborn baby. In other words, evoke positive changes in yourself so you can be the best husband and dad you can be.

If you can't make an emotional investment now, then what makes you think you will do it after the baby's birth? Because so many men don't follow through, they destroy their relationships with their children. Do you want to spend the rest of your life repairing or building a relationship with your eventual child, teenager, and adult?

If you still think a man isn't capable of expressing that much passion for fatherhood, visit and chat with a seasoned at-home dad in your community. Despite having their masculinity questioned and labeled with names like "Mr. Mom," bum, and loser, this population of men has proven that a man can overcome social ignorance and embrace fatherhood with the same kind of passion and commitment that a woman does with motherhood. At-home dads have also proven that they can fulfill the role of primary caregiver just as well as at-home moms can.

Ask any at-home dad I know, most of whom had well-paid professional careers, and they'll tell you that their decision to become the primary caregiver was one of the best decisions they've ever made in their life. None of them feel that they sacrificed their careers. In fact, they believe they traded their careers for something better—time with their children. It was a conscious decision they've never regretted.

One father who still hasn't regretted his decision from two decades ago to be an at-home dad explained: "The original plan was for me to stay home with our two kids until they entered elementary school. But I fell so in love with being an at-home dad that I'm now into my twentieth year."

If a man can embrace and express his commitment and passion for a sport or hobby, he should be capable of doing the same for an unborn baby. If you don't embrace fatherhood, not only will you miss out enjoying life with the baby, but you will also fail to reach your full potential as a dad.

One of the best compliments I received during my work with expectant dads came from a wife. She telephoned and said, "Thanks for giving my husband the courage to be an involved dad."

I hope you will open up your heart and find the courage to embrace fatherhood.

— 22 —

Make peace with yourself about your father

— 22 —
Make peace with yourself about your father

I want to make it perfectly clear that this chapter is not about you making peace with your father but making peace with yourself about your father. Whether you decide to personally resolve your issues with your dad or forgive him is up to you.

During the introduction in the expectant dad classes I conduct, I invite the dads to talk about their fathers. Keep in mind that most of these men haven't formally met each other, yet they feel comfortable sharing intimate and painful details about life with their fathers. And that is because I ask the dads to present their stories in a nonjudgmental, noncondemning way. Of the thousands of dads who have attended, only one has turned down my invitation.

The purpose of the exercise is to help each dad come to terms with who his father was and move on with his life as a new dad. Whether your dad impacted you in a negative or positive way is not as relevant as how it will affect the way you embrace fatherhood and father your children. Let me share my personal story, one that has often been repeated by other dads but with a less positive outcome.

I'm a product of a divorced family. A single working mom raised me. My mom never talked about my dad, Henk. I never asked about him because I thought it better that I didn't bring him up. I had resigned myself to the fact that I would never meet him. Well, I was wrong—fate brought us together twenty-seven years after he had last seen me.

Unlike most men, I had built up no animosity toward my dad. I was not looking for retribution or an apology. I was just happy for the chance to meet Henk.

He told me his side of the story, and I discovered that the decision to divorce and move to another country was my mom's. He tried to contact us, but my mom's family would not cooperate. He went on to apologize for not trying hard enough to locate me and also for not being around during my childhood years. I accepted his apology. As he was crying, I realized that he had missed me more than I had missed him. From that point on, I had an awesome father-son relationship with Henk until the day he died.

Not all absent-dad stories turn out in a positive way like mine did. I know many men who have never forgiven or made peace with their fathers. But that was their choice. I feel sorry for these men because I experienced the benefits of reconnecting with my father. One thing I know is that I'm at peace with myself because of the effort I made to repairing my relationship with Henk. And finding peace within you is not about how the story ends but the emotional investment and effort to make amends.

Not having a dad physically around is painful, but not as painful as a dad who is emotionally absent. My heart goes out to all the men whose dads were in the house but were emotionally distant. It had to be very painful walking into a house with a dad who didn't care enough to spend time with you and be there when you needed him.

One of the most heartwrenching stories I have heard about an absent father came from a teenager whose dad was an alcoholic and drug addict. He was asked what he would say if his dad were sitting in front of him now, and he replied, "Why were drugs and alcohol more important than me?"

At the other end of the spectrum are new dads who have shared wonderful stories about their fathers. Fathers who were great providers, did a good job balancing work and family, helped with the housework, and spent time with their children, regardless of how tired they were after work. The challenge for a new dad who grew up in this situation is the pressure of filling his father's shoes.

There are other new dads who have been victims of sexual and physical abuse. I'm not an expert in dealing with these kinds of situations, nor have I experienced them. I'm sure it must have been devastating. However, if a new dad doesn't address or come to grips with his past or seek professional help, he can wind up just like his father.

As you can see, the family dynamics of each father, good or bad, is very broad. All of us have some painful emotional baggage, and what is in your baggage differs from the baggage of others. But it's not about the baggage, it's about how you deal with it. So many new dads despise their fathers yet model the same behavior. The choice is up to you. Do you want to keep going through your life as a new dad carrying the unhealthy baggage that might destroy a relationship with your new baby? Or do you want to break the cycle and stop the generational curse of being an emotionally distant dad?

I made the commitment to be an involved dad for two reasons: one, because I didn't want my children to experience life without a father the way I did, and two, because I never wanted to experience the painful emotions Henk felt the day he regretted not being in my life, and miss out on spending time with my children.

My father was not perfect. I'm not. No one is. There is one thing I know, though: that there is always room for improvement. And I realized that I couldn't make improvements as a father if I didn't make peace with myself about my father.

– 23 –

Learn more about your wife's father

– 23 –
Learn more about your wife's father

S tudies show that there is a direct link between a daughter's relationship with her father and her perception and choice of a man. The studies also show how the father-daughter relationship will affect a woman's behavior once she is in a committed relationship with a man. Researchers believe that father absence has as much an effect, if not more, on a daughter as it does a son. If that is the case, then there should be more cause for concern as to how unresolved issues a new mom has with her father can negatively affect the way she perceives and treats her husband and father of the unborn baby.

Most dads don't recognize the warning signs and dysfunctional behavior a new mom may begin exhibiting due to her father's absence, and the few dads who do feel awkward addressing the changing dynamic in the marriage. The conditioned response for these men is to hide in their man caves. This head-in-the-sand approach creates only more conflict with no resolution in sight. As I noted in Chapter 17, this is another situation in which you need to speak up. Don't abandon a new mom in this time of need by being emotionally distant like her father was. Help her face and overcome her fears about your role as a new dad.

Most new moms have a tendency to be overprotective, possessive, and overbearing about their new role as a mom. Women, by nature, experience mood swings when they are not pregnant. Add pregnancy in the mix along with the unhealthy baggage a new mom carries from her relationship with her father, and her actions and behavior can undermine your efforts to be an involved dad.

Here is a list of possible inner conflicts your wife may struggle with and not discuss with you. Be aware that almost every woman doesn't want to share intimate details about the strained relationship with her father for fear that her husband may also abandon her.

A daughter who had a strained relationship with her father or one that involved emotional, physical, or psychological abuse may lack the confidence and the rationale to recognize the value and role you play in the pregnancy. She may also question her confidence and ability to be a good mom. Therefore, this is when you as a new dad will need to demonstrate some compassion with words of encouragement and assurance that you will not abandon her.

A new mom who has unresolved issues with her dad may also fear that her husband will inherit her father's incompetent or abusive behavior and eventually turn into her father. She may expect more out of her husband to ensure that he doesn't follow in her father's footsteps. She may purposely create unnecessary conflict because she had to endure it with her dad, so without conflict, her life as a mom will not feel normal. She may be uncomfortable when her husband undertakes a more emotional and nurturing role because it was the complete opposite of her father and therefore may cause her to view his behavior as "unmanly." She may focus on a new dad's shortcomings rather than his strengths and effort to be involved because of her father's ineptness and inability to follow through. This can lead her to criticize a new dad for not doing enough. She may not encourage a new dad to be involved to protect her from reliving the many disappointments she experienced with her father.

If a new mom's father was controlling, she may interpret her husband's enthusiasm as a power move to control and dominate her life as a new mother, which may lead her to hinder a new dad's efforts to be more involved during the pregnancy.

These inner conflicts a new mom may have can lead her to unknowingly and unintentionally act out behaviors that will sabotage rather than strengthen the new family bond a new dad is striving to create.

Here is an example of a scenario that describes how a new mom can be encouraging one moment before the pregnancy and then discouraging at another time after the birth.

In Chapter 13 I noted how a new mom encouraged her husband to attend the expectant dad's class offered at the hospital. After the new dads graduated from the class, I invited them to return with the baby six to eight weeks after the birth to be mentors for the new corps of expectant dads who attend future classes. Very few accepted the invitation, and I was curious to know why. So I conducted a telephone survey and discovered that the main reason the dads didn't return to class with their child was the new mom's reluctance to relinquish and entrust the baby to dad.

A daughter who had a good relationship with her father develops a constructive sense of confidence, assertiveness, and stability. These positive traits help a daughter become more secure and confident about her role as a mother as well as your ability to be a good dad. If your wife falls into this category, consider yourself lucky. However, there is still cause for concern.

With a good father in her life, a wife may expect her husband to live up to her father's billing. The high expectations and pressure to live up to dear old dad may set a new dad up to fall short or fail. It is unhealthy for a wife to make a comparison between her husband and father. Likewise, a new dad must also be careful not to make a comparison between his wife and mother.

I'm not suggesting that a new dad pry into his wife's relationship with her dad or help her heal the emotional wounds and make peace with her dad. That will be her decision. What I am suggesting is that you as a new dad become aware of your wife's state of mind to help resolve any future conflict, and also to help your wife be the best mom she can be.

— 24 —

Encourage your wife to accept a dad's perspective

— 24 —

Encourage your wife to accept a dad's perspective

Almost every new mom is infatuated with her pregnancy, and rightly so. Not only is it an exciting time, but it is also overwhelming with all the physical changes to her body, mood swings, and social pressure. Furthermore, childbirth instructors and solicitations from parenting magazines bombard moms with the notion that it is all about her and the baby. Hence, moms have very little patience, time, and energy left to think about what their husbands think and feel about being a new dad.

At the same time, moms also expect their husbands to learn and read about what mothers experience during a pregnancy. Yet rarely will moms make time to read any book on fatherhood to gain more insight on a dad's perspective. I know this from personal experience and also from a survey I conducted in my workshop for moms.

In the workshop, I asked the moms two questions. "How many of you expect your husband to read books on motherhood?" They all raised their hands.

"How many of you have read a book on fatherhood?" None of the moms raised their hand. (I didn't accept a book on pregnancy that had a section or chapter about a father's perspective.)

You might find a few exceptions in which the mom has read a book on a father's perspective. If she has, it paled in comparison to the number of books a new mom expects a dad to read.

Tina and I have been married for twenty-one years and she still hasn't read a book on fatherhood. All these years she has only viewed and lived parenthood from a woman's perspective. Needless to say, life with her has been a challenge because of her narrow view. Unlike most men I didn't hide in my man cave or give up on finding ways to help her overcome her ignorance on the subject.

Communication with a woman isn't one of a man's greatest strengths. Nevertheless, if I can manage to persuade my wife to accept a dad's perspective on parenting, any new dad can also do the same with his wife.

What I learned from my experience with Tina is that the key to unlocking the close-minded view a mom has about pregnancy and parenting is to learn how to communicate in Venusian. It's that whole "Men are from Mars, Women are from Venus" thing. The strategy here is to talk like a Venusian in order to help your wife think and view pregnancy like a Martian.

I know what a new dad might be thinking: Why can't I tell it like it is? Why can't I say what I feel? I feel the same way, but as I noted in Chapter 6, don't let your EGO prevent you from accomplishing your main objective—to help your wife see and accept a dad's perspective.

A straightforward, logical, simple conversation does not always work with a woman, especially a pregnant mom who is emotionally unstable. Discussing the what, how, and why of a situation sounds rational but it doesn't necessarily compute with a woman. What does work is building rapport, nurturing the conversation, and understanding how you feel about a situation before getting to the point. For a woman it is not about the solution but rather learning more about how you feel and not what you want her to do. Once she knows how you feel, she'll be more likely to show more compassion toward you and accept your perspective.

I'm not suggesting that you show your feminine side because men don't have one. What I am suggesting is to change how you speak and deliver the message to your wife. My rule of thumb is that if my wife doesn't understand what I've said, then it's up to me find a different way to communicate so that she understands.

I'm careful not to just blurt out what I feel or let my emotions get the best of me. Tone of voice and posture is also important to control. At six feet six inches, I can be very intimidating, so I make sure that I'm sitting down. I also have a loud voice, so I had to learn how to tone it done. And finding the right time to have a conversation is vital. I try to make sure that Tina isn't experiencing one of her mood swings when I approach her. If I sense she is, I will ask her when it will be a good time to talk. Relinquishing control to her made her feel I was less of a threat. The latter does require some self-control and patience. Sometimes I will also write down what I want to say to Tina because she doesn't handle person-to-person conflict very well, and a letter is also less threatening to her.

Here are some do and don't examples of how to express to your wife any frustrations you may have. In print is what a new dad is likely to say, followed by a more appropriate way to share these thoughts (in italics).

Why are you spending all this money? Will you please stop? We're going broke. It doesn't make any sense to buy something just because it's on sale.

Honey, when I see the credit card bill at the end of the month, the message I get is that I need to work longer hours and make more money, not spend more time helping you at home.

Why do I have to keep going to these childbirth classes with you? All the childbirth instructor talks about is stuff about you and the baby. It's boring. There are other things I'd rather be doing.

Honey, I've attended six childbirth classes with you to learn more about your pregnancy. And last weekend I attended a class for expectant dads. If a class for moms about a dad's perspective is available, will you attend the class?

Geez, not another book to read! How many books are you going to make me read? I don't have time for this.

Honey, this is the fourth book you've asked me to read. I've learned a lot about what you're going through. When I was at the expectant dads' class, a dad suggested I buy you this book on fatherhood. Will you read it for me? It will really mean a lot to me if you do.

Why does the childbirth instructor keep calling me "coach" and "partner"? I'm tired of the political-correctness crap. Why don't you say something to her?

I noticed that the childbirth instructor is always referring to me as "coach" or "partner." She makes me feel like I'm your assistant and not an equal partner. I'd prefer she call me "dad" because I'm proud of my commitment to you and the baby. Would you mind saying something to her?

Why can't you accept my point of view? Why does it always have to be your way or the highway? You're not the expert just because you're carrying our baby.

Honey, I've heard you say many times that you want me to share how I honestly feel about something. But each time I do, my comments seem to have no credibility or value, or you get upset at me. Can you see why I sometimes clam up and hide in my man cave? What man wants to continue getting his head cut off each time he opens his mouth to give his honest perspective?

A new dad's goal should be to communicate to become closer to his wife and help her understand how he really feels as a new dad. His goal shouldn't be to get her to understand what it's like to be a dad because she can't, just like a man will never be able to understand what it is like to be a mom.

~ 25 ~

A new dad never loses the title of Dad

— 25 —

A new dad never loses the title of Dad

My commitment to each of my children is no different than the one I made to my wife in our wedding vows. I'm their dad for better or for worse, for richer or for poorer, in sickness and in health, to love and to cherish, until death do us part. Never did this vow reign more true than in the case of our second son, Wesley, who was born with a rare genetic disorder.

Once a couple decides to have a baby, they have no control over the genetic make-up, sex, personality, or outcome of the baby's health. Mom and dad are at the mercy of nature. The baby is nonreturnable and theirs forever. Although each birth is a life-changing experience filled with great expectations and dreams, not all dreams parents have for their children come true—few children turn out the way parents had hoped. Despite wishes for a bright future with a healthy child, there are no guarantees.

One of the top concerns a dad has is the health of the baby. The thought of what might happen is always in the back of his mind. No matter how hard a dad tries to think it away, there are times when the pregnancy or birth doesn't go well. It is the natural order of life, and nothing can prepare a new dad to deal with news of an unhealthy baby.

Wesley's birth in 1989 was just as special as the birth of our firstborn, Grant. The words "It's a boy" brought great joy to me for the second time. But for the next few weeks, Wesley experienced medical complications. A few months later joy quickly turned to sorrow after I received the following words from the doctor: "Mr. Hilling, your son Wesley was born with a rare genetic disorder."

The doctor didn't use the word disabled, but I sensed that the dreams and life I imagined living with Wesley had come to an abrupt end.

The news of Wesley being disabled for life—that he could not talk or walk and would require 24/7 care—tore my heart and shattered the dreams I had of life with him. While each dad deals differently with the news, most dads cannot cope or come to grips with accepting and loving the baby unconditionally because in their eyes, giving birth to a disabled child is a sign of failure. For these dads, the baby is considered damaged goods. The macho manhood mentality leads most men to abandon the baby or divorce his wife. A few dads, however, do find the spiritual strength to march on and fulfill their duty as fathers. I feel fortunate to be one of the latter.

I'm not here to judge or condemn those dads who have decided to abandon their disabled baby. Many dads have done so with a "normal" baby and regretted it. What I am here to do is to demonstrate that a man never loses the title of Dad.

After a brief mourning period, I had a personal revelation inspired by the 1990 movie *Awakenings*. The movie's tagline is "There is no such thing as a simple miracle." The plot is that victims of a encephalitis epidemic many years ago have been catatonic ever since, but now a new drug offers hope of reviving them.

The next day I decided to put the sadness behind me and rethink my perspective on fatherhood. I came to several conclusions. I decided not to let the disability define Wesley and accept him for who he is. Wesley was the one who was disabled, not me. I decided not to allow his disability prevent me from honoring my duty as his father.

My simple miracle with Wesley was not to fix him. In my eyes he wasn't broken. Wesley's disability was not an act of God but of nature. Some people suggested I pray to God for a cure. I decided that it wasn't fair to make that request because then God would have to fix all the disabled children.

Although I had lost the initial dreams I had envisioned with Wesley, I realized that I could make new dreams with him. The evening after watching *Awakenings,* I made a pact to live up to Wesley's expectations of me as a dad and wrote the following poem titled "Instead" as a guideline for my life with him.

Instead of walking with you, I will crawl with you.
Instead of talking with you, I will find ways to communicate with you.
Instead of isolating you, I will create adventures for you.
Instead of focusing on what you cannot do, I will focus on what you can do.
Instead of feeling sorry for you, I will respect you.

Wesley is now twenty years old. Just as with my two other boys, I have fond memories of life with him and no regrets about having him as my son.

I hope he is just as proud to have me as his dad.

− 26 −

Help your wife adjust to motherhood

— 26 —
Help your wife adjust to motherhood

One day your wife is just a married woman, then after a passionate night of love-making with you, she becomes a mom and you a dad. Once a woman announces her pregnancy, it will require her to make some adjustments, just as she did after she agreed to be your wife.

Although people experience changes throughout their lives, nothing is more dramatic than the transition from wife to mom. And no wife can prepare herself for the changes she will inherit as a mom.

While many women choose to become mothers for its rewarding nature, they don't understand how intense, how emotional, or how difficult it is to be pregnant until it happens. The transition into motherhood can be very overwhelming and challenging as it requires a woman to adapt to the physical changes in her body, reexamine who she is as a person, and explore and navigate the unfamiliar territory of being a new mom.

The first and most obvious adjustment an expectant mom experiences is her physical appearance. A woman is under incredible social pressure to maintain a certain body figure even during pregnancy. Every time a pregnant mom enters a grocery store, convenience store, or drugstore, she is bombarded with magazines containing photos of celebrity pregnancies that paint a glamorous lifestyle most expectant moms cannot afford. The media reporters neglect to mention the available time celebrity moms have to exercise and the available money for personal trainers, healthy food, and in some cases, postpartum plastic surgery. The reality is that most expectant moms will struggle with weight gain.

A new mom will also experience an overwhelming sense of responsibility and feel guilty if she can't fulfill all of her obligations. (By the way, working dads also feel guilt for the same reason.) As a wife, she had a busy life with a career and managed to juggle a list of chores, duties, activities, and projects. After a typical working day, she came home and had time to cook dinner, relax on the couch, watch television, and not worry about anybody else but her husband. She also had the luxury of an active social life that included dates with her husband, parties with friends, and weekend trips. Suddenly, as a new mom she will lose some of her freedom and acquire other obligations like baby showers, doctor visits, childbirth classes, writing and mailing thank you cards, and so on. With more on her plate and less time and energy, she may feel discombobulated and disorganized.

In addition to nurturing a marriage and family, today's new mom is also expected to nurture a successful professional career. Some moms may have fears about the reactions of their employers or clients: How do I announce my pregnancy to my boss? How will my coworkers feel about the special treatment I may receive from the boss? Some may have concerns about how the pregnancy will affect their performance: How will my coworkers, employer, or clients react to any delays on projects caused by my pregnancy? Some may worry about losing their balance and falling: How do I deal with safety concerns at work? Some may struggle with finding the right time to take maternity leave: If I submit a maternity leave request too early, how will it affect my position when I return to work?

As you can see, an expectant mom has a lot to be concerned about during her pregnancy. Because most expectant moms don't accept and follow advice from their husbands very well, the strategy here is to provide reminders that will help your wife adjust to her role as a new mom. Keep in mind that some expectant moms may need reminders more often than other moms do.

Remind and reassure your wife that you still love her, and tell her what she means to you. A constant display of affection with hugs, flowers, cards, or words of comfort will help her overcome her insecurities about the weight gain and make her feel loved. If your wife is working outside the house, send the card or gift to her place of work. The attention she will receive will boost her image and self-esteem and also score huge brownie points for you.

Remind her that it is okay to ask for help and delegate duties to other people, as discussed in Chapter 14. Help her build a support network for herself. Don't let her play the guilt card either—she doesn't have to play "Super Mom" and do everything herself. Remind her to take care of herself by eating healthy food and resting when she is tired in order to recharge her battery.

Remind and encourage her to mingle with other expectant moms. Don't let her isolate herself. Remind her that you don't expect the house to be as clean as it was before the pregnancy. Remind her that when people ask her to volunteer or invite her to a social event that it's okay to say "no," or at least tell them she needs to consult with you before giving an answer. Women have a tendency to say "yes" because they feel obligated or want to avoid the guilt trip that accompanies saying "no." Overscheduling can place a lot of stress on you and her as a couple, so help her maintain a good balance.

Finally, remember that an expectant mom can get so caught up in the challenges of motherhood that she forgets to enjoy it, so remind your wife that becoming a mom is a cherished experience to enjoy and share.

– 27 –

A new dad's transition into fatherhood is tough on everyone

— 27 —

A new dad's transition into fatherhood is tough on everyone

While you are struggling to adjust to your role as a new dad, so is everyone else in your social circle and working network. With all the attention and focus on mom's priorities, people overlook a man's transition into fatherhood and don't express the same courtesies to a new dad as they do to a mom.

People are quite aware and in tune with the physical and emotional adjustments a woman experiences when she becomes a mom. They understand the science behind a woman's weight gain and the overwhelming responsibility a woman has in carrying a baby in her womb because she is the lifeblood for the baby. There is also a level of sympathy and compassion a woman receives that isn't offered to men.

The reality is that most new dads struggle with their new status in a world ignorant of the transition into fatherhood. People don't realize that a man's adjustment into parenthood is just as complicated and complex as a new mom's. Even though today's new dads have been more involved than those in the past, studies show that people still feel uncomfortable and out of place with a dad's presence and involvement. And that is because our culture has not taught either women or men how to embrace fatherhood in the same way they do motherhood. This lack of concern about a new dad's transition can induce even the most confident of men to surrender or neglect their duties as new dads, which divorce and separation statistics have shown happens far too often.

Dads, however, have also contributed to this ignorance because they struggle to make the difficulties of their transition common knowledge. Instead of tackling the issue of transition, men often resort to hiding it under the rug. Well, ignoring it will not help and will place added stress on your marriage, affect your performance at work, and influence relationships with other people in your life.

A new dad doesn't have to be shackled by his and other peoples' ignorance. Instead, a new dad can accept the responsibility of educating people and encouraging them to extend to dads the same courtesy, respect, and treatment they offer moms.

A new dad may think he is coping well with the transition but might come across to his wife and others as uncaring and uninterested. Or people might interpret his behavior as though nothing is wrong, that he is coping well with his new role. And then he will interpret their behavior as heartless and unconcerned. The end result leads to unresolved conflict, and nobody benefits.

Regardless of whether it is comfortable to do so, a new dad needs to openly address and discuss with others the adjustments he is making and must make to become a father. As I noted in Chapter 13, people can't help with your transition into fatherhood unless you speak up and tell them what you need. Don't be shy. When the opportunity arises, let people, especially your wife, know how you are struggling to adjust to your identity as a new dad, what is bothering you, and what they can do to help resolve the anxiety and stress you feel.

There are so many misconceptions about men as fathers, but one of the truths about fatherhood is that people in general don't know how seriously a man plans to take on his role as a dad. Therefore, it is up to you to show people how serious you are about it.

Some of the transition issues you as a new dad may encounter include adjustments to the relationship with your wife, relatives, friends, coworkers, and employer, as well as your priorities, work schedule, spending habits, and overall lifestyle. The sooner a new dad makes the adjustments, the sooner he will be able to enjoy his life as a new dad.

If a new dad's wife pressures him to attend all the doctor's appointments, and his coworkers and employer share their unhappiness about taking too much time off of work, he must let her know about it and discuss some options. When you approach your employer, take responsibility by outlining a plan to resolve the situation. The employer will appreciate your initiative and be more likely to compromise. This may sound risky, but you stand to lose a lot more if you don't speak up.

If you have a conflict with a relative or friend, deal with it immediately. He or she may not understand how important it is for you to be a hands-on dad, and you may not have conveyed it well enough. Both of you may feel that your friendship is in jeopardy. And you don't want to lose relatives or friends because they will become a source of support. A friend or relative may interpret your constant answer of "no" to invitations or offers to help as cutting off ties with them. When you say "no," follow it up with an explanation and encourage them to keep inviting and asking. It's important to keep the lines of communication honest and open.

Here is how you can help yourself and others with your transition and in turn, earn their respect.

Announce to everyone, including your employer (make sure you give enough advance notice), that you will be taking two to four weeks off after your baby's birth, utilizing the Family Medical Leave Act or your vacation time. I highly recommend a staycation for every new dad because of the following benefits. First, it gives you a significant amount of time to bond with your new family and help you focus on the job you have ahead of you as a dad. Second, you'll get a chance to hone your skills as a caregiver. Third, you'll develop empathy for your wife in her new role as a mother. Fourth, it will give time for you and your wife to learn how to work together as a team.

Just like you, the people around you are also entering your world of fatherhood blind. Since you're the dad, be their guide and help them help you transition smoothly into this important role.

– 28 –

Establish a work-family balance schedule

— 28 —
Establish a work-family balance schedule

One of the toughest adjustments most new dads struggle with is balancing work and family time. How much time do I devote to family without jeopardizing my job? How much time do I devote to work without jeopardizing the relationship with my wife and new baby? How can I fulfill all my obligations as an employee and new dad and still balance both? What kind of lifestyle do I want for my new family? How can I make the most out of the time with my wife and new baby? Many dads have a difficult time coming up with solutions. Some never do and end up neglecting their new family.

This issue can become such a burden that most new dads will usually allow work to take precedence over the wife and baby and rarely succeed at finding the right balance between work and family. This is because their masculinity is defined by their profession and how much they earn—not by how much time they spend with their family. Throughout my young adult life and before the birth of my first son, nobody addressed or taught me how to balance work and family time.

Like all young boys, I was raised with a deep sense of obligation to my role as a financial provider. The number one priority was establishing a professional career. The second was the almighty dollar. I spent a majority of my time hoping to live the American dream of owning a house with the white picket fence and relying on my future wife to take on most of the responsibilities of raising the children and managing the household because that is the way our culture said it was supposed to be.

Another ongoing struggle about balance is peoples' misconception of what "balance" actually means. Balance in respect to work versus family time is not about equal time or making up for lost time. It is about establishing a reasonable ratio between a dad's time at the office and at home that works best for his family. There is no one-size-fits-all solution to balancing work and family.

A schedule that works for one family will not work for another because of their different professions and dynamics. For example, a salesman who travels a lot will have a different work-to-family-time ratio than a UPS employee, a doctor different than a teacher, a police officer different than a stockbroker, a fireman different than a store manager, and an accountant different than a janitor working the graveyard shift.

There are also not enough hours in a day to equally share time at the office and work. Let's break it down. Out of twenty-four hours, a third is spent sleeping. That leaves you with sixteen hours, eight to ten of which must be allotted to work. Then you have to subtract three miscellaneous hours for meals and unexpected situations, which leaves you with only three hours a day to devote to family time and managing the household. That gives you a ratio of about 5 to 1 of work-to-family time. Therefore, if you work a forty-hour workweek, a good goal to shoot for is eight hours a week of family time, which includes helping out with household chores. That breaks down to about two hours per weekday. I did not factor the weekend hours because you will use them as make-up hours. For example, if you decide to use an hour of alone time on Wednesday evening, then you should make up an hour of either family or household chore time on Saturday or Sunday.

How you incorporate this balance ratio into your schedule will be based on your profession and the lifestyle you choose to live. If your profession requires you to work more than forty hours, at least come up with a reasonable ratio and make up for other hours on the weekend. If you decide to be the primary caregiver or work part-time, then you have more flexibility. Use the 5-to-1 ratio as a standard to work with, make adjustments along the way, and hold yourself accountable to whatever you choose.

If your employer pressures you to work more, then defer to what I've suggested about outlining a game plan. If your employer is not willing to compromise, you still have options. You can take a stand and seek legal advice, interview for another job, or make a career change. There is no reason for you to work in a job that is going to negatively affect your new life as a dad. I've heard too many horror stories that resulted in divorce.

Once you establish a schedule, stick to it. It is important to be consistent. Then implement your game plan as soon as possible during the pregnancy. Live during the pregnancy as though the baby is there. Make some test runs. Plan out days to leave work early to help you and your employer adjust to your new lifestyle. Once you arrive home, help out with the household chores. You and your wife should already have a "who-does-what" list.

The next important thing is that work should not get in the way of family life. Separate the two and keep work at work. Don't let the job control your family life because doing so will only lead to distraction. The same applies to bringing family issues into the workplace, which can impair your productivity.

You can also apply the ratio strategy to household duties that you and your wife will split. Again, forget about equal division of labor. It doesn't exist. One of the spouses will always take on more of the workload.

Balancing work and family will also require a lot of trial and error and periodic analyzation of what is or isn't working. Like marriage, finding the right balance that works best for your family will always be a work in progress.

– 29 –

Schedule reasonable "me" time

$-29-$

Schedule reasonable "me" time

Parenting is the only profession in which a person will not have regular time off. At your office or place of work, it is a given that you will receive time off for lunch and a morning and afternoon break to reenergize your body and mind so that you'll perform better. Most employers recognize that an overworked employee is less productive and at risk to harm himself or other employees. The same is true with parenting.

Life was hectic enough as a husband. Now that you're a new dad, you'll be asked to juggle even more life issues and take on more responsibilities in the same twenty-four-hour period. The days add up to weeks and to months, and you still haven't taken a break. You feel obligated to honor requests from your wife, employer or client, parents, other relatives, and friends. Trying to fulfill all of them is taxing, and you can't keep plugging away without a break because you'll wear yourself down physically and emotionally. Not taking care of yourself is bad for you, your wife, and the baby (I refer back to the airplane oxygen mask analogy).

The reality is that you'll never have enough time in a day to accomplish everything you set out to do, or resolve every challenging issue that comes your way. So why fret over taking time off to escape the rigors of life for an hour or two? Whatever issues or projects you had on your list before you took time off will still be around after you spend some quality time alone.

Alone time is one of the most unused and under-valued aspects of parenting. Most parents, especially moms, don't recognize the significance and benefits of "me" time, so they don't utilize it. They also view alone time as a selfish act. Most moms even allow guilt to keep them from taking a short break. The truth is that new dads and moms should allow themselves to view alone time as a deserving reward.

Experts say that "me" time is a basic need, whether it's solitude or with people other than your wife. I know you love your wife, but time away from each other is healthy. The way I look at it is that I need a break from my wife as much as my wife needs a break from me. (You'll also find this to be true with children.) With the busy world we live in and all its distractions, it's easy for a man to fall off the daddy track. The alone time will help you clear your head so you can refocus on keeping your priorities as a new dad in tact.

For some, being around others can be exhausting, so these people need solitude. Others hate being alone and need the social contact. Whichever you choose, you simply need "me" time to recharge your mind and body—even if it's just for one hour. "Me" time is a great stress reliever and also gives you freedom to rest and not worry about the next deadline or project. It's also an escape from having to impress or gain approval from someone. It's a time just for you to relax, calm frazzled nerves, and have no worries.

One fear a new dad may have is selling "me" time to his wife. It's okay to request alone time from your wife as long as it's reasonable and you give equal alone time to her. If you have a wife who won't utilize "me" time, don't let her hold it against you when you use it. Just because she doesn't want to take alone time doesn't mean you shouldn't. Once you come to terms with an equitable arrangement, be consistent in blocking out "me" time on your calendar. It's important to establish a consistent ritual so your wife knows not to schedule any appointments or social events during that time.

An hour or two of "me" solitude time per week is reasonable. Some ideas for private time include going for a short walk or jog, working on a hobby, working out at the gym, reading a book in a hammock, hitting baseballs at a batting cage, and reclining to watch a television show or movie. If you're an early riser, wake up an hour earlier. If you're a night owl, ask your wife to block out one hour before bedtime.

A social activity with your friends once a month is also a reasonable request. Some ideas include poker night, a drink at a bar (make sure you get home safely), pick-up basketball games at a gym (not a league), volleyball at the beach, or a tennis match at a park or club.

An example of unreasonable requests includes eighteen holes of golf, softball league, bowling league, or any social activity that involves more than four hours at a time or a weekly commitment. With respect to golf, you can't justify spending eight hours on any activity. A compromise in this situation would be to play only nine holes of golf, either the front or back nine. With respect to softball and bowling leagues, you can serve as a substitute and play once or twice a month. If you're currently involved in weekly social activities, it's important to gradually scale down as soon as possible. Life after the baby will not allow you to keep the same schedule.

It's okay to be good to yourself. You don't have to give up your entire social and active life when you become a dad. With the right attitude and support from your wife, you can manage to find time for yourself and also be a great husband and dad.

─ 30 ─

Network with other dads

― 30 ―
Network with other dads

As an entrepreneur, I understood the importance and value of networking in the business world. The personal interaction with other businesspeople created opportunities to market my service, raise my profile, drum up new clients, access free information, and engage in brainstorming sessions. But in 1991 when James May introduced me to the networking concept for dads, I questioned whether it would work because I didn't see the value in it and wasn't convinced that other dads would accept the concept. As you can see, I didn't demonstrate much faith in my fellow dads.

I understand firsthand how unnatural and uncomfortable it is for a man to accept the idea of attending a networking group with other dads. It is as unnatural as a man admitting he is wr . . . wr . . . wr . . . not right or asking for help. But that shouldn't serve as an excuse for dads not to give it a try. As Benjamin Franklin said, "He that is good for making excuses is seldom good for anything else." It also doesn't mean men aren't capable of embracing the concept of networking with other dads to discuss father-related issues.

Since that eventful day in 1992 when I became an advocate for fatherhood, thousands of dads through programs like NFN (National Fathers Network), FNOC (Fathers Network of Orange County), and BCND (Boot Camp for New Dads) have proven they can network with other dads. These dads have also demonstrated that if a dad can make time to hang out and network with other dads at the lodge, bar, golf course, tennis club, casino, or sporting event and have discussions about sports, business, politics, television shows, movies, and glory days, there is no reason a dad can't make time to meet and talk about fatherhood. These dads also showed that, just like moms, they could juggle time between fatherhood, career, and networking with other dads. It all boils down to a matter of priorities and making the time.

New moms instinctively connect with each other and comfortably share their hopes, fears, and shortcomings about motherhood. As your wife's pregnancy progresses, be aware and understand that she may choose to confide with female friends and relatives because they can empathize with her. If your wife questions your intent to network with other dads, remind her that it's important for you to also huddle with other dads for the same reason she does with other moms.

If you're still reluctant and can't overcome the fear, remember the advice I gave in Chapter 13: you're not alone! Unfortunately, most dads' misconceptions about hanging out with a bunch of dads to talk about fathering issues is no different than peoples' misconceptions about men as inept dads.

To help you feel more comfortable about a dads' networking group, let me first describe what it is *not*.

What it is not: It is not therapy, a touchy-feely or lecture-based session, or a step program. It is also not a forum for politics, religion, medical issues, or parenting philosophies. There are plenty of professional organizations that provide these services.

What it is: It is a forum for exchanging information and ideas on fathering issues among dads. What separates the networking concept from the other fatherhood programs and makes it unique is that the dads—not the organization or pundit—control the agenda and content of the forum. Boot Camp for New Dads is a prime example.

As I mentioned in the introduction to this book, I was hired in 1994 as a consultant and instructor for Boot Camp for New Dads (BCND). The program encourages expectant dads to attend the class before and after the baby's birth. What makes the class unique is that graduates from the program return with their babies (six to eight weeks old) to mentor the new attendees. New dads not only get the benefit of learning from other new dads but also the chance to handle a newborn. One lucky dad even gets to change a diaper. You can find BCND in hospitals across the country and learn more about their program and locations at www.bootcampfornewdads. org. There are also other independent expectant dad programs available. Check your local hospital or community service center for more information.

Here is a list of guidelines to help you determine how a dads' networking group should operate.

The network should:

- Provide a safe, nonjudgmental environment.
- Respect privacy and establish the following rule: No quote that identifies a dad is shared outside the network without his permission.
- Encourage dads to help each other become better husbands and dads for their families.
- Only address and discuss issues related to fatherhood.

- Assign a designated facilitator whose only job is to manage the open-discussion forum. The facilitator does not have to be a health care professional. Any dad can fill this role as long as he has had the proper training.
- Allow the dads, not the facilitator, to choose the topics for discussion.

A formal networking dads' group should meet once a month. A $15 to $25 fee per meeting or yearly membership is reasonable, especially when you compare it to other activities men spend money on—like a $100 to $200 round of golf. A typical dads' network meeting is two hours, but oftentimes the meeting takes longer, and that is okay. The meeting should begin with a brief introduction by the dads, followed by at least ninety minutes of open discussion, and end with the facilitator inviting the dads to share one thing they learned from each other.

If you still struggle with attending a dads' networking group, invite another expectant dad or male friend to attend with you. Or better yet, invite your father or father-in-law as some other dads have in classes I've facilitated. Another way to feel comfortable is to pretend you're heading to the locker room to talk with a bunch of guys about the sport or topic of fatherhood.

If there is no networking dads' group in your area and you would like to start one, you can contact me to learn how through the Daddyshome, Inc. Web site at www.daddyshome.org, and click on the Speaker's Bureau icon.

Networking doesn't just have to be in a formal group setting like BCND. A new dad can also network with other dads in his neighborhood, church, and place of work. The number of dads you network with is not important. What is important is that you're networking.

A new dad can also go virtual and join one of the fatherhood Web sites that have discussion forums. If you are one of the dads who is uncomfortable in a person-to-person setting, the Internet is a great place to start. However, be careful not to isolate yourself. At some point a new dad should ease his way into networking person-to-person with other dads, or he will never reap the true benefits of networking.

Once you decide to take the same leap of faith that I took in 1992, you'll discover the following benefits:

- *Validation.* You will meet other dads who feel the same way you do. You will realize that you know more than you think you do and that your perspective on parenting matters.
- *Recognition.* You will discover that your instincts as a father are legitimate. If your wife disputes an opinion you have, the group provides you with credibility.
- *Knowledge.* You will have access to free information and resources from the shared experiences provided by the other dads.
- *Camaraderie.* You will meet and develop a common bond with other new dads, each aspiring to be the best dad he can be.

- *Support.* You will increase the number of people in your support system and reap the benefits listed in Chapter 14.
- *Self-assurance.* You will boost your confidence in your ability to perform your dadly duties. That confidence will help you minimize mistakes and conquer the challenges of fatherhood.
- *Valor.* You will provide courage to each other to be a hands-on and involved dad.
- *Mentorship.* You will have other dads to look up to who will help you stay on the daddy track. Together you will inspire each other to improve your fathering skills.
- *Fulfillment.* You'll gain the satisfaction of knowing that you helped another dad and will eventually become a mentor for another new dad. You will feel valued and help other dads feel valued as well. But more important, your involvement will make networking an accepted practice for your son or son-in-law and future generation of new dads.

Once you decide to take the leap of faith to join a dads' network, it is very important that you approach it with the right frame of mind. First, set aside any presumptions of what to expect from sitting with a group of dads to have a serious discussion about fatherhood. Second, a dad's value to the group should not be measured by how much he talks. Many dads need to develop a comfort level before breaking out of their shell. This may be the first time one of the dads has experienced this type of forum and been invited to voice his opinion about being a dad. If you are one of these dads, how much you talk or share with the group isn't as important as being there. You're presence itself is important to the whole networking group. You'll soon find your comfort zone, and when you do, your contribution to the networking group will stand out. Third, don't sell yourself short. You will soon discover that you know more than you think you do. Fourth, don't underestimate the value of your role as well as the roles of the other dads. Each of the dads brings value to the group.

Fifth, the value of networking is not about the information shared among the dads but rather about the camaraderie and the relationship-building process that comes with it. As your relationship with other dads improves, so will your relationship with your wife and new baby. Sixth, remember that you're in the group to help and support each other.

The extent to which you (and the other dads) benefit from networking will depend on your commitment and can only be measured by how much time you invest. I highly recommend that you continue networking with other dads after the baby's birth because the best resource a dad has to become a better husband and dad is other dads.

Check out these other books in the
Good Things to Know series: